GW00858504

If I Can, You Can

Research: Sarah Chapman, James Morgan, Katerina Smith, Gregory Blackman and Olivia Cartwright.

Edited By Jacqueline Rose

Published by Lovely Silks Publishing 2016

If I Can, You Can

This book is presented solely for educational and entertainment purposes. The author and publisher are not offering it as legal, accounting, or other professional services advice. While best efforts have been used in preparing this book, the author and publisher make no representations or warranties of any kind and assume no liabilities of any kind with respect to the accuracy or completeness of the contents and specifically disclaim any implied warranties of merchantability or fitness of use for a particular purpose.

Neither the author nor the publisher shall be held liable or responsible to any person or entity with respect to any loss or incidental or consequential damages caused, or alleged to have been caused, directly or indirectly, by the information or programs contained herein. No warranty may be created or extended by sales representatives or written sales materials. Every company is different and the advice and strategies contained herein may not be suitable for your situation. You should always seek the services of a competent professional.

If I Can, You Can

If I Can, You Can

There have been many twists and turns, challenges and setbacks, but with each one I have kept pushing forward, and facing so much adversity has helped me become who I am today.

Les Flitcroft

I'm not the brightest or best at what I do (there will always be someone better than you, I learnt that lesson a long time ago), but there will only ever be one best you.

Claire Curzon

Don't be the doubter; there are enough of them anyway. If you can find it in your heart to be the one who shares hope, it will raise your spirit too. Be the hope carrier you would like to meet.

Alex Couley

Many people are self-destructive without even realising it, because they are consumed by negative thoughts. These thoughts are repeated so much that they can become a self-fulfilling prophecy.

Sarah Jones

If I Can, You Can

It's amazing what the mind and body can do when you have something you really want to achieve.

Anjay Zazulak

I have no idea where it came from but a voice within said "I'm going to recover, I'm going to get better and I'm going to make sure this *never* happens to anyone else!"

Sarah J Webb

8 | P a g e

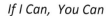

Living with HIV can empower you to even greater ambitions. My HIV has made me the person I am today.

Philip Christopher Baldwin

If someone who faced the prognosis of a persistent vegetative state can get published in a book aptly named "If I can you can"then imagine what else might be possible if you fire your imagination.

Lisa Beaumont

My dad said to me "you remind me son of one of the students I have just expelled. He told me he likes to do well, but he doesn't want to do well".

Luke Hughes

When one learns to ask the right questions, the right tools magically appear and that's when we become the master of our own Destiny.

It worked for me and if I can you can.

Leann Middlemass

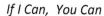

Back then, I wished every morning that I woke up that I hadn't. But I never lost the spark of hope that I could get better.

Carly Evans

The inspiring people that have contributed to this book:

Claire Curzon

Carly Evans

Leann Middlemass

Sarah Jones

Les Flitcroft

Lisa Beaumont

Alex Couley

Sarah Webb

Helen Johnson

Philip Christopher Baldwin

Anjay Zazulak

Luke Hughes

Table of Contents

Welcome to If I Can, You Can

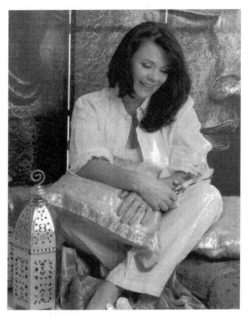

Nowadays many of us live life in the fast lane and rush from one week to the next, often just getting on with our own daily routines. Some of us just about balance looking after those nearest and dearest to us and occasionally manage to find time for ourselves. Many of us simply feel we haven't the time to give much thought for others, not only in our immediate communities but the world in general.

Just once in a while we may read an article that helps us realise that there are people battling against all kinds of odds just to make it through each day. Then, perhaps we stop to give a thought of empathy. It is at that time we thank God that whatever they're going through, won't ever happen to us or our family. And then we move on. And there are those people that always stand out as they are always smiling, totally selfless, and thoughtful, making the world a better place.

Within these pages of If I Can, You Can we will be sharing personal stories from contributors from around the globe. Our writers are from very different walks of life. And yet the common theme in all their stories is the fact that life has presented them some incredible challenges. Some have been faced with near death experiences but, with the support of family, friends and their communities, have fought back to find a new path in life. A path that is better than the one they were originally on. Even though some of us plan the journey of our lives meticulously by achieving set goals within a scheduled time frame, we sometimes find that, due to incidents we hadn't foreseen or expected, we are way off course.

I hope that by showing how others have managed to overcome their challenges, If I Can, You Can will provide you with the confidence and faith you need face your difficulties. Often when we overcome obstacles thrown at us by life, we begin to appreciate the true value of life and all of its gifts. It is then that we can truly move on to live life to its full potential.

Jacqueline Rose

Publisher, Lovely Silks Publishing

Pranic Healing

I've experienced more tragedy than you could ever imagine possible for an average man who was once content just to lead an ordinary life.

There have been many twists and turns, challenges and setbacks, but with each one I have kept pushing forward, and facing so much adversity has helped me become who I am today.

It's been an extraordinary journey...

Let's roll the clock back to 1999, the year my life hit a brick wall. Literally.

I was competing in an indoor football game when I tripped and was catapulted straight into the wall of the sports hall where we were playing — with catastrophic results.

Some of the details of what happened next remain hazy as I was in so much pain, but it quickly became clear that I'd shattered the bones in both my arms and this was serious. Just how serious only emerged after five major operations and countless hours of rehab: my doctors told me there was nothing more they could do for me, and I would never regain the use of my left arm.

Bad enough for most people, but I am left-handed and I worked as a hands-on aircraft engineer.

Life couldn't get much worse — except that it already had. One of the reasons I was in that sports hall in the first place was to escape, to try to find a way of temporarily distracting myself from something much, much more devastating, something truly traumatic: a year earlier my estranged wife had committed suicide after suffering depression for nearly five years, taking our two young children with her. They were aged just seven and five.

It is hard to put into words a tragedy of this magnitude and for others to grasp the impact it has. It is fair to say that I'd had many moments in the months that followed when all I wished for was to join my family — I only stopped myself because of the thought of the further devastation it would bring to my parents.

I had already hit a virtual brick wall long before I hit the real one.

While I was in hospital after the accident I became very depressed, as all I could do was lie there thinking of what had happened in my life. My left arm was in a harness, paralysed, and my right arm was plastered above the elbow. I had needles in both feet — one for pain relief and the other for antibiotics — so I couldn't move at all.

I had four operations in quick succession (the final one came later) and each time as I went down to theatre I remember saying to the nurse standing next to me that I wished and prayed I would not wake up again. I had come to the end of what I thought I could deal with, but still I kept waking up to carry on the fight to survive.

When I finally left hospital after two weeks, I had to think of new ways to distract my mind and thoughts: it was a constant battle. Somehow I'd hung on and hung on, only to now find myself facing the loss of my livelihood as well.

I had always wanted to be an aircraft engineer. Some of my earliest memories of growing up in my home town of Reading in Berkshire are of playing with model aircraft and dreaming of one day being able to work with the real thing, being able to fix them.

My career in engineering started in the oil and gas industry, manufacturing valves for subsea pipelines, but in 1990 I joined British Airways. I ended up working at London's Heathrow and continued my career in aircraft engineering for more than 20 years, also working for Hawker Pacific Aerospace and Lufthansa Technik. My childhood dream had come true, and even if my personal life was in desperate tatters by the time I smashed into that wall, I was well on the way to achieving all I'd set out to do professionally.

Until the doctors told me my left arm was permanently paralysed. They'd pinned it, they'd put screws in it, I'd had every type of physio on offer, and while the bones had healed to some extent, the nerves were severed at the elbow. Severed forever, they said.

You don't need to be a genius to work out that there aren't many options for a left-handed aircraft engineer who can't use his left arm and by now I was nearly two years down the line from that fateful day in the sports hall.

My employer had been supportive all the way, but time was beginning to run out and it's fair to say I was pretty desperate. I just couldn't see any way out of this nightmare, and so when a friend suggested I explore energy healing I figured anything was worth a try.

Before I go on, it's central to my story to know a little more about where I've come from. My father is ex-Army — he was a sergeant — and you'd be hard pushed to find anyone, anywhere who sees life as more black and white than he does. When my brother and I were growing up, we naturally enough adopted our dad's world view that there simply are no grey areas — in anything. He had no time for religion, for anything spiritual, for anything you couldn't see, touch, hear, taste or smell. Sceptical doesn't come close, and that may be one reason why I was so drawn to becoming an engineer: you can't get more black-and-white than fixing aircraft. They either fly, or they don't fly!

So, coming from this background, you can see that the very idea of exploring energy healing for my arm took me way, way out of my comfort zone. I knew nothing about any kind of complementary therapy — I'd vaguely heard of treatments like osteopathy, acupuncture, and maybe even Reiki, but as far as I was concerned this was all woo-woo nonsense. You were injured or ill, you went to the doctor.

But desperation triggers all kinds of responses, and in my case it was to conclude that with all conventional medical avenues now closed, I had absolutely nothing left to lose.

So in 2001, I found myself travelling to the United States to meet my friend and to join a Pranic Healing training course. I'd done a little bit of research before I set off, and knew that this was a non-touch therapy that used natural energy to heal. Non-touch? Natural energy? You can imagine how well that played with my black-and-white sceptic's outlook.

As we settled into the course, I was doing my best to keep an open mind and soon became fascinated by what the man who went on to become my teacher and mentor was saying. This was Master Choa Kok Sui, who developed modern Pranic Healing and introduced it into the public domain in 1987 from his native Philippines.

What caught and held my attention — and continues to do so to this day — was the logic and structure underpinning Pranic Healing. Master Choa was himself an engineer, and his whole approach was something my pragmatic brain could quickly grasp. This wasn't woo-woo at all, it was science-based and from the start of the course we were being encouraged to validate everything we did.

For every condition, there was a protocol, a means of removing stale and unhelpful energy from the body and replacing it with fresh energy — or Prana, the Sanskrit word for life force. All we needed to do was follow the protocol, clearly spelled out, in writing, by Master Choa — I immediately likened it to a cookbook approach: simply follow the recipe, don't deviate, and see what happens.

And what happened to me was nothing short of a miracle. My friend introduced me to Master Choa and — despite my being just one of more than a hundred students on the course — he took time out to show me the specific protocols I needed to heal my arm. He was so concerned by my plight, and so generous with his time — I remember it all as if it were yesterday.

I began following the protocols Master Choa had taught me straight away and continued after I returned home, healing myself studiously for 20 minutes every day. Within a few weeks I was aware of some feeling returning to my arm; within five months I was completely healed. In just those 20 minutes a day I had achieved what I'd been told was completely impossible: all the nerves in my arm had regrown. Now all that remains of that horrendous ordeal are some very impressive scars!

Not surprisingly, I wanted to find out more about Pranic Healing — how it worked, how I could use it to help other people. It's taught in stages, and after I'd completed the basic course I returned to the US to take the more advanced classes, one of which was the psychotherapy course which focuses on the mind and emotions. This helped me in so many ways to understand why people become mentally ill and gave me much insight into my late wife's illness and the tragedy that I had faced. My respect for Master Choa grew and grew each time we met and when he said he wanted me to be the one to take Pranic Healing into the UK and Ireland, I knew I'd reached a major crossroads in my life.

I was by now back at work as an aircraft engineer, and Master Choa insisted I do nothing to jeopardise my source of income in the short term. So for ten years, I led something of a double life, juggling my demanding day job with building my Pranic Healing practice, teaching others how to heal, and spreading the word slowly but surely.

From simple coughs and colds, cuts and bruises, right through to cancers, depression, addictions and phobias, I was soon healing a wide range of people from all walks of life. Babies, children, young and old, my experience of extreme pain— both mental and physical — gave me a good understanding of other people and how they felt when confronted with the conditions or problems they faced.

Among my early clients was a five-year-old boy with a brain tumour. His parents had been told there was little hope for him, but by working alongside conventional medicine I was able to use Pranic Healing to help disintegrate the energy within the cancer cells and he went on to make a full recovery. I also treated a paramedic signed off for over a year after being diagnosed with post-traumatic stress disorder. He was able to drive again after his first session, and was back at work as a front-line responder after just seven treatments.

And the successes kept on coming.

Despite all this evidence — and even remembering what I'd witnessed with my own arm — I still had many moments when I asked myself 'did I really do that? Or was it something else?' It was just my black-and-white engineer's mind-set jumping in — and it was this that also explained why for several years when I was healing I couldn't feel the energy.

I've since found that many people who attend Pranic Healing courses — especially if they've come from sceptical, analytical or atheist backgrounds — put exactly the same obstacles in their own way, and I always reassure them that it is just a matter of time. And — as I'd already demonstrated so clearly — it doesn't stop you getting spectacular results.

In 2013, I finally left engineering behind and became the director of the Institute of Pranic Healing UK and Ireland. It is of course much, much more than a job, or even a profession. Pranic Healing isn't just about healing the body; it's also about healing the mind and developing spiritually, and Master Choa's system includes meditations and practices drawn from across many traditions to help us all achieve this, to help us all have a better life. As time has gone on, many of my students have followed in my footsteps and also become full-time healers after experiencing extraordinary results for themselves.

One of them is also now among my team of instructors, training new students so we can reach and help more and more people. He had come to the end of the line with traditional approaches when he first found Pranic Healing. He'd been diagnosed with the rare Kleine-Levin Syndrome sleep disorder at the age of 16, and for a period of five years he had slept for five days in seven.

He was introduced to me by his previous employer, and by the time I met him he was in his early 30s and had explored complementary as well as conventional avenues. He had made some progress, but despite doing everything 'right' — eating well, exercising, studying personal development, practicing moderation — he remained so debilitated by severe anxiety and other psychological and emotional issues that he couldn't work for long periods without having to take time out to sleep.

After his first treatment he began to experience some relief from his symptoms, and after several more his symptoms rapidly diminished and then disappeared altogether. He began to feel healthy for the first time in more than a decade, not only physically but also emotionally and psychologically, and he soon decided that as well as following his dream and building a career as a personal trainer, he had to share what he had discovered with others.

His is just one among many examples of how Pranic Healing can transform lives, and since I accepted Master Choa's invitation to become his ambassador more than 2,000 students have graduated from my Pranic Healing courses in the UK alone. There are many hundreds more in Ireland, as well as in Gibraltar and Spain's Costa Del Sol, and together we have healed many hundreds of thousands of people. Together we also host more than 200 meditation and healing clinics every month. Here we use a mix of meditations, including Master Choa's very powerful and effective Meditation on Twin Hearts which pivots around the Prayer of St Francis of Assisi and its focus on using loving kindness to turn negatives to positives.

I personally teach over 30 courses a year as well as continuing professional development sessions for my core leadership team, which is growing stronger every year. I also host monthly lectures and meditations, which are open to the public and are streamed live to multiple locations across the UK and Europe. And I also still have my own healing clinic, based in Berkshire.

One of my strongest passions is helping the next generation grow up into happy, balanced young adults, and among my proudest achievements is creating a children's meditation programme. This is now being used in British and Irish schools, with some extraordinary results.

It has been truly humbling to see the quality of life for thousands of children — among them those with learning disabilities, autism, and other complex psychological and emotional challenges — rapidly improve as a result of simply following the meditation techniques. I am also very proud of the wider contribution to the community being made by the Pranic Healing charities, the MCKS Charitable Foundation UK and The Association of MCKS Ireland. All donations made at our meditations, healing clinics, and other events go to these organisations, which in turn donate to other carefully selected charities.

Between the UK and Irish charities, we have donated considerable sums of money to many organisations such as Crisis and the Whitechapel Mission for the homeless in London, and the Naomi House, Richard House, and Alexander Devine children's hospices. Other beneficiaries include Doctors without Borders, HOPE suicide prevention centre, and TeenLine Ireland.

When I look back to when I broke my arms in that sports hall wall and then look at where I am today, I am amazed by what I have achieved and what it is possible for us all to achieve if we stay focused, work hard enough, and keep going despite all the odds.

On the personal front, my remarkable journey also has a happy ending. In 2008, I married my beautiful wife Fiona, and we are now the proud parents of three wonderful children. My aim for the future is to continue what Master Choa Kok Sui started, helping relieve unnecessary suffering and teaching people that everyone deserves and can have a better life. To this end, my personal mission statement is 'to help alleviate suffering by empowering people with self-development tools through support, educational programmes and charitable services to create healthy and resilient communities' — something I could never have imagined the skeptical aircraft engineer stating in public a decade ago!

Les Flitcroft

*"Every day is a new day,
a day that you have never experienced before
and will never experience again.
Enjoy it as if it was the last day"*

About The Author

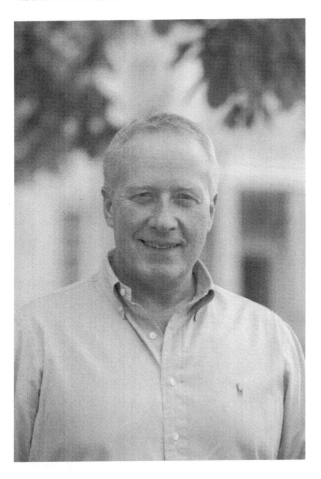

Les Flitcroft is the Director of the Institute of Pranic Healing UK & Ireland and a former aircraft engineer who discovered this energy-based complementary therapy following a serious sports accident.

After achieving life-changing results for himself, he has gone on to devote his life to Pranic Healing and as senior instructor for the UK, Ireland, southern Spain, and Gibraltar, has already trained several thousand others to become Pranic Healers.

He is the founder of two associated charities, the MCKS Charitable Foundation UK and The Association of MCKS Ireland.

www.ukpranichealing.co.uk

https://www.facebook.com/UKPHealing/

https://twitter.com/pranicuk

https://www.instagram.com/pranichealinguk/

Happy, Healthy and POSITIVE

Cold. The floor was icy cold. I pulled my knees into my chest. I made myself breathe slowly. I did not want anyone to hear me. I wanted to be invisible. I wrapped my arm around the side of the toilet. My watch scratched along the limestone floor. Safe. I wanted to feel safe. I rested my head on my arm. The wool of my jacket nuzzled my neck. It felt reassuring. My loafers were pressed against the locked cubicle door. I had checked several times that it was locked. I wanted no one to find me. I could smell bleach. My face rubbed against my sleeve. I wanted to be clean. I desperately wanted to be totally clean.

I looked at the curve of the toilet bowel. I ran my index finger along its ceramic form. I tapped its side with a neatly filed fingernail. The rhythmic motion was reassuring. I started to feel the cold of the floor in my hips. My arm was getting stiff, my contorted bicep hard beneath the cotton of my shirt. The condensation of my breath warmed my chest. I strained my wrist to see the time. I had been there fifteen minutes. I had to return to my desk.

I was diagnosed with HIV in January 2010, when I was 24 years old. I visited Birmingham the morning of my diagnosis for a business meeting and rushed back to London to attend the sexual health clinic. I wanted Post Exposure Prophylaxis (PEP). This can be administered within 72 hours of possible exposure to the HIV virus to prevent transmission.

At the beginning of the appointment I was told that I needed to take a blood test to ascertain my current status. I was tested in the spring of the previous year and believed myself to be HIV negative. About thirty minutes later the nurse summoned me into a consultation suite to give me the news. The room was large and empty, except for some seating and bland posters. The blinds were down and the room was full of afternoon shadows.

I sat in a chair with my back to the wall and the nurse sat opposite. She was in her mid-forties, slightly overweight and with streaks of grey around her temples. It was a complete shock to learn that I was HIV positive. I was speechless. I struggled to breathe. I was overcome by an aching anxiety. I turned my head to one side and looked at the floor. The nurse tried to engage me in conversation, asking what I was thinking. She gave me some basic information on HIV and informed me of the next steps. I tried to take in what I could. I was sitting on my hands, to try to stop myself panicking. I breathed slowly, but wave after wave of anxiety washed over me.

The nurse left the room and I was alone. I tried to compose myself. I wonder how many times she had told someone that they were HIV positive before.

I hid the news from my colleagues upon my return to the office that afternoon. I avoided conversation and tried to appear occupied with emails. I left early. I was in a state of confusion. I made my way to the gym. I did not want to stop being a muscular young man. The next morning, with a mounting sense of apprehension, I made my way to the office. It was difficult dealing with the platitudes of colleagues at work. They chatted about the weather and their quiet evenings at home. There was a surreal moment as I ascended to the fourth floor in the lift.

My employer's London office has a large central atrium with six glass panelled lifts. The lift was unusually crowded. I squeezed in, smiling politely at those either side of me. One was reading City AM, a financial newspaper, and a few were checking their Blackberries. They were bathed in normality. I was battling the emotional turmoil of having been diagnosed with a petrifying illness. I wanted to cry, shout and scream.

I sat at my desk for a few minutes, before hiding in an adjacent office. I closed the door. I turned my body inwards, cocoon-like, trying to suppress my sadness, guilt and fear. I broke down. Tears welled up in my eyes. I did not want anyone to walk in and find me crying, requiring an explanation and potentially resulting in the discovery of my HIV. I wrapped my arms around myself, my hands gripping the ridge of my back. Swaying backwards and forwards I sat on the edge of the desk. Legs crossed, my body was contorted with pain. I pulled my arms inwards, my forearms pressing against my stomach. I felt dizzy. I retreated to a corner. I pressed my head against my knees and looked at the wall.

The next week, running up to my initial appointment at the HIV clinic, was one of fear. I wanted to learn more about HIV, its potential impact and what my options were regarding treatment. My uncertainty was heightened by the pressure I was under to conceal this from my employer. I was concerned my career would be damaged. I knew of no one working in financial services who was openly HIV positive in the workplace. I tried to distract myself with the routine of work.

My identity as a talented and ambitious gay lawyer was being undermined. My life seemed to have lost a large part of its meaning. I stumbled through, as in a daze. I took the morning off, lying and saying that the medical appointment was in relation to the removal of a mole. I wished I had the confidence to tell my supervisor about my HIV.

My friend Anthony came with me to the HIV clinic. It was in an unfamiliar part of London. I had only been to Whitechapel once before, when I had briefly dated a guy who lived around the corner from the tube station. The taxi pulled up outside the hospital. The Royal London Hospital is a large Victorian edifice. I rummaged through my pockets for the appointment letter, which included instructions on how to locate the clinic.

The Grahame Hayton Unit is situated at the rear of the building and took us a while to find. We waited at the reception, before being taken through to a second waiting area. The consultation room was smaller than the one at the sexual health clinic. Windowless, but brighter. With Anthony, myself and several nurses, the space felt crowded. It seemed slightly claustrophobic. I sank into an armchair. I unfastened a cufflink and rolled up the sleeve of my shirt. My composure slipped when a trainee nurse struggled to find a vein, missing eight times. In the middle of the consultation I was informed that I was not only HIV positive, but also co-infected with Hep C. My heart plummeted. Ten minutes earlier the same nurse had reassured me that HIV was completely manageable, but had warned that I needed to be careful not to become Hep C positive. My ears went numb. I could no longer hear what was going on. My stomach felt as if it was lined with lead. I wanted to curl up and cower.

Anthony took me to a cafe, buying me some sugary food. I was tired and lethargic on account of the vials of blood, which had been taken. I had a slice of lemon loaf cake and a hot chocolate. I ate slowly, gradually returning to some normality. I prepared myself to return to the office. I can remember little of that afternoon. Of course I did not tell my colleagues where I had been, and what for. I kept up the pretence, behind, which I echoed with deafening emptiness. I was in silent agony.

A grey day had turned into a dark evening. It was bitingly cold outside. I dislike January. I was wearing a heavy wool coat over my suit, but it was not keeping me warm. My dad had bought the coat for me from Harvey Nichols in my final year at school, five years earlier. I am very careful with my possessions and treasure items, especially when they have memories attached.

It had been a stressful Wednesday in the office, although I was relieved to escape work relatively early. I was not looking forward to catching up with my mum. The previous week's events had taken their toll. I felt listless, physically tired and emotionally drained. I still wanted to hide myself away and nurse my wounds.

I sat down at a circular table in the back of the restaurant. My mum was late. A cute Italian waiter asked me if I already know what food I wanted to order. I eat here regularly. I explain that I am waiting for another diner. Just a diet coke for now. Candles flicker atmospherically around the expanse of the darkened restaurant. Large cast iron columns support a wood panelled roof. Neatly piled pastries adorn the front of the restaurant. Laughter at a neighbouring table upsets me. I bite the inside of my mouth, chewing my lower lip and running the tip of my tongue over my teeth. I can taste blood.

I look up. I think I can see my mum outside the restaurant. She seems to be loitering. I am unsure if she is on the phone, or maybe she is having a cigarette. I thought cigarettes supressed the appetite. I tap my loafer against the wooden chair leg, in time with the background music. She pushes the door, a long shadow sweeping the entrance as it opens. Slowly she climbs the steps. It is my mum. She stands there, looking slowly around the room. She is carrying a fabric bag over her shoulders. The weight seems to be dragging down her slight frame. My mum is very beautiful. She has blonde hair. She is in her fifties, but looks much younger. People occasionally ask if she is my sister.

The Italian waiter bends over the neighbouring table, distracting me. They have just settled the bill and he is thanking them. There are flecks of grey in his beard. My mum has seen me. She walks up the left side of the restaurant, pulling her bag upwards and looking to either side. She is accosted by a waitress, who greets her with flamboyant gestures and a smile. My mum purses her lips. She squeezes past another table. I look up at her and smile.

Thirty minutes later I am home again. It had been a very short meal. I am upset. I had forgotten my mum's birthday, which was on the previous Friday. She was angry. I had noted her birthday in my diary, but it had completely slipped my mind. My mum is not a lady who minces her words. She can be very direct. She is understandably hurt. She said that I am cold, distant and selfish. Her admonitions were hard to deal with, each one wounding me. Did I do it intentionally? Do I not love her? Why do I care so little for her? I am protecting her. I cannot tell her the truth about my HIV diagnosis. I need compassion, reassurance and love. I love my mum so much.

My diary from 2010 has the usual flow of social engagements, gym appointments and increasing work commitments. I was trying to hang on. I wanted my life to be as normal as possible. I increased the number of training sessions that I did with my personal trainer. I wanted to prove to myself that I was healthy. I trained rigorously.

My career continued to progress well. I had great supervisors and enjoyed the work. I felt I could not tell my supervisors about my HIV either, or confide generally in the workplace. Few people are comfortable disclosing their HIV status in the workplace and certainly not in investment banking, at international law firms, large accountancy practices, or other City institutions.

There is a fear their careers will be irreparably damaged and that assumptions will be made about their sexual behaviour. I did not want to place colleagues in an awkward position and had to make excuses to attend medical appointments. I was not ashamed of being HIV positive, but being furtive about my HIV in the workplace reinforced the sense of stigma I experienced. Lying about my HIV was diminishing me as a person. This made it much harder for me to come to terms with my diagnosis. The stress of concealing my HIV status had a substantial detrimental impact on me.

I had to juggle hospital appointments with taking on new career challenges. I moved from the corporate department into capital markets, the area I would ultimately specialise in. In April 2010, I spent a week in Brussels, learning more about my employer and the opportunities which were available to me. I compartmentalised the emotional pain and uncertainty. I tried to stay focused on my work. I was determined not to let my HIV diagnosis impact my career.

I told Stephen, my best friend at work, who was also gay, about my HIV status. He was supportive, but I did not have the confidence to tell anyone else. I was creating solid foundations for my career, but there was also an element of denial in my defiance. My emotions were contained within a dam. The floodgates were firmly shut. At work, I was unable to open up to those around me about my HIV.

In June of that year, I attended a team building weekend with the department. A lot of my colleagues brought their partners. I would have felt comfortable bringing a boyfriend, as the environment was inclusive. I was petrified about my colleagues discovering my HIV status though. I felt as if I was at school again. I had grown into an out and proud gay man, after years of LGBT bullying at school. I had become so confident in my sexuality. I now had a new secret. I was furtive around my HIV status. I had to deal with a massive amount of self-stigma. I was petrified of how my colleagues would react. My life became a mire of paranoia. I was evasive about my health. I responded with platitudes. I shut myself off from my colleagues.

Summer had turned into autumn. The photographer was arriving at 7.15 pm, with the guests expected at 7.30 pm. They were kind at work, letting me leave at 5 pm, so that I could get ready. I am wearing my favourite red Alexander McQueen jacket, a grey vest and blue jeans. This is an important night for me. I have arranged a dinner for fourteen people as part of the Terrence Higgins Trust Supper Club. The purpose of the dinner is to raise funds and awareness for the THT, the UK's largest HIV charity.

I am hosting the dinner at the One Aldwych Hotel, in a private room. Before the dinner we are doing drinks in the Axis Bar. I have invited my closest friends, who have supported me through this difficult time. It is ten months since my HIV diagnosis. I am in the middle of a crazy deal and have been working every weekend. My employer was supportive of me taking the evening off, because I have been putting so many hours in. I told them that I felt compelled to organise the dinner as part of my LGBT activism. No one guessed that I was HIV positive.

We are going to do photographs in the main bar, on the sweeping staircase down to the restaurant and then in the private room. I reviewed the menu with the restaurant's maitre' d' the previous week and co-ordinated the seating plan. Two large bouquets of flowers have been placed where we are going to dine. They have printed menus and place cards. The room looks beautiful.

Joe, Luke, Anthony and Francis, my three closest gay friends, are all here. Joe was the first person I told about my HIV diagnosis. I thought my world was about to cave in. I called him, on the evening of the day of my initial diagnosis, after I returned from the gym. He was reassuring, telling me that everything would be ok. He pointed out that there are incredible treatments, meaning that HIV is not a death sentence now. We spoke on the phone for about an hour. I went to bed feeling more composed.

I told Luke the following morning. Luke was shocked, but supportive. I had taken a course of PEP a year earlier and, at the time, we had a long conversation about the treatment. PEP lasts a month and there were extensive side effects. He said, back then, that I should not throw my life away. The day after my diagnosis, I felt as if this is what I had done. I called Anthony to tell him about my HIV a few hours after Luke.

Anthony has a number of friends who are HIV positive. I did not know any HIV positive people myself. He told me that my life would not change that much. Later that day, Luke and Anthony chatted, Anthony agreeing that he would come to my first appointment at the HIV clinic with me.

Francis was amazing. We sat in a restaurant, a few days after my initial diagnosis and he said that he would also introduce me to some of his HIV positive friends. He said he would always be there for me. I could not have got through this period in my life without my friends.

My mum was looking glamorous in black. In the initial weeks, following my diagnosis, I thought I might tell her, but then I took the decision to keep my HIV a secret from her. I am petrified of hurting her. I want to shelter her from the truth. I think this is the right decision. She is really enjoying herself this evening, which pleases me. I know that she wanted to meet more of my friends and this seemed like a great opportunity.

My friend Marc, who has hosted for the THT before, gave a really moving impromptu speech, congratulating me on a wonderful evening. I was very touched. I sat between Luke and Joe. I glanced at my Blackberry a few times, to check my work emails. Looking back at the glossy photos now, one of which is framed on my bedside table, it is hard to grasp the fear that I was experiencing during my first year as HIV positive.

I was seconded to the NYC office in 2011, a time of great excitement. I noted the one-year anniversary of my HIV diagnosis in my diary. I referred to it cryptically, not specifying the occasion. I was worried in case I lost my diary and someone found out that I was HIV positive, or in case it fell open on that page and a colleague guessed.

My employer had offices in over thirty countries. Some of the international secondment destinations, like Singapore, had mandatory blood tests for HIV.

In principle Singapore bans foreigners who are HIV positive from entering the country. A blood test is required for any foreign national staying longer than 30 days. Those with HIV face deportation and doctors are obliged to alert the authorities.

My mum wanted to take me out for dinner, in February 2011, before I flew to NYC. I had seen my HIV and Hep C specialist the previous day. He said that it was ok for me to go to NYC. We had a long conversation about how my life should never be limited by my HIV status. Because of my Hep C, I had four appointments a year with my specialist, rather than the usual six-monthly HIV check-up. He said that it was no problem for me to spend six months in the USA, as I was so healthy. There was no possibility of my developing any health complications related to my HIV whilst I was abroad and he gave me his personal telephone number, which reassured me, in case of any unforeseen circumstances.

I ran my hand over the soft fabric of the seat, savouring its texture. My right leg was comfortably crossed over my knee, the white table cloth curving over my thigh. A pleasing diagonal fold ran up the centre of the table. The starched linen felt like canvas. I was relaxed. I had a steak, as well as side portions of spinach and green beans. My mum was enjoying her salmon. My mum has a slight appetite. I love eating out with her because I normally get to eat half her food. My mum was having a glass of wine. I was not drinking anything at all then, on account of my Hep C. My mum, of course, knew about neither my HIV or Hep C at this time.

I had explained my sudden decision to stop drinking alcohol by saying that I was on a detox. The lie slipped from the tip of my tongue. I had then "enjoyed" my detox so much, that I decided to continue with it. My mum believed this and said that I had even inspired her to go on a detox. I do not like lying. I did not feel guilt about not telling my mum the truth about my HIV and Hep C. I was hurt emotionally about my HIV. I was trying to come to terms with it myself and at this stage I did not feel comfortable sharing my HIV status with my mum. I was wounded. I was entrenched. I felt that I could deal with the pain on these terms. My terms.

I had some sort of control around it. At least I could control who I disclosed my status to. I had my own boundaries and I had to be really comfortable before I was able to push these. I was scared the fear would otherwise ricochet outwards. And potentially overwhelm me.

The apartment my employer had rented for me was a few blocks away from the trendy Bowery area. I could not wait to see it. I was very lucky that I would be living in Manhattan. My mum was flying out with a friend to visit me in March. She was really pleased that my career was going so well. I had five days to settle in, before I started at my employer's NYC office. I already knew which gym I was going to join. My friend Francis had told me to train at the David Barton gym on Astor Place.

My six months in NYC were an incredible time. In a number of ways this was the most exciting period during my 'twenties. I travelled to Washington, Miami, Boston and Montreal. I was working like crazy, but also wanted to see as much of the USA as I could while I was there. My HIV was lurking in the background, but I did not have to confront it yet. The USA had changed their immigration policy in 2010, meaning that HIV positive people no longer had to declare their status when applying for a visa. This was a big step forwards for equality. I felt welcome in the USA!

In mid-May my friend Joe travelled to NYC to visit me. He stayed at the apartment my employer had rented for me. I could not take any time off, as I was working on a huge deal, which was set to complete the following month. In the evenings we had a chance to catch up and savour the City. My birthday, which is on 22 May, fell during his stay. It was a Sunday, but I was so busy with work that I had to be in the office all day.

I escaped for a few hours in the evening for dinner. I held the alabaster candle holder in my hands. The candle inside flickered gently. I placed it back on the table. The light shone evenly through its striations. It cast an orange glow. No shadows. I had rushed downtown and it was great to hang out for a few precious hours with Joe.

Upon my return to London, as an associate, I specialised in bond issuances. I did long hours, but enjoyed the quality of the work. At the end of 2012, my CD4 count plunged, triggering a period of depression. It was at this point that I told my mum I was HIV positive. She was very upset. She was worried I was going to die. I managed to partially reassure her. I suggested that she meet my HIV and Hep C specialist, which helped massively.

After initial infection patients are not treated with antiviral medication until their CD4 count falls to around 350, some people remaining healthy for up to ten years before their CD4 count falls and antiviral medication is required. I managed three years, which is about average, going on Truvada, ritonavir and

Darunavir in January 2013. This was a difficult time for me, but having the support of my mum helped greatly. The medication is highly effective and within a month of beginning treatment the physical decline in my health was reversed.

I finally told the partnership and HR about my HIV at the end of 2012. It was the uncertainty surrounding the fluctuation in my health, which led me to confide in them. From the beginning of 2013, I was completely open in the workplace about my HIV status.

Telling my employer, and to an extent my mum, was an empowering process of acceptance, a second coming out as important regarding my identity as coming out as gay had been a decade earlier. Coming out as gay in my teens allowed me to develop my gay identity and gain acceptance around who I am. Telling my colleagues about my HIV empowered me, enabling me to incorporate my HIV fully into my identity.

It took me several years to come to terms with my HIV diagnosis. I was one of the first people working in the City, at either an investment bank, international law firm or major accountancy practice to be openly HIV positive in the workplace. Stigma surrounding HIV remains very real and HIV visibility is a real issue, especially in the workplace where there is often a reluctance to talk about this. Confronting HIV stigma is a core part of my human rights agenda.

Speaking openly about my HIV and Hep C is one of the most important things I have done. My activism and charitable work are now the main emphasis in my life. I am proud to describe myself as a gay rights and HIV awareness activist. Helping others is the most wonderful and empowering feeling in the world. Importantly, by talking about my own experiences, I can hopefully challenge some of the stigma, which exists today about living with HIV. My HIV diagnosis was one, which was at first frightening, but this has come to transform my life and empower me. I am a healthy, happy and successful HIV positive man.

My HIV does not hold me back. I progress ever forwards, my life improving as I become more confident in who I am. I have taken ownership of my HIV status, incorporating this into my identity. My HIV has made me a stronger person and I do not believe that I would be the person I am today had it not been for my diagnosis. I went through a process of becoming more open, allowing myself to be reborn.

I forged a new identity, enabling me to become a different person from either a high-flying gay lawyer or a terrified patient. My humanity and humility was deepened through the experience of being made vulnerable and humbled. A weakness became a strength. It is our flaws, which make us beautiful. My HIV undermined me, leaving me vulnerable.

Now it is a core part of who I am. My experience of coming to terms with my HIV diagnosis caused me to grow as an individual. I am full of hope and optimism for the future. I have now left my job in the City to pursue my activism.

At the heart of this is the struggle against HIV, both nationally and globally. I would like every person to know that they can overcome the uncertainty of an HIV diagnosis, that those living with HIV can have an incredible life, full of hope. Living with HIV can empower you to even greater ambitions. My HIV has made me the person I am today.

Philip Christopher Baldwin

About The Author

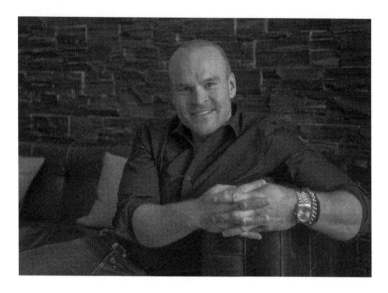

Philip Christopher Baldwin is a gay rights and HIV awareness activist. He studied History at Oriel College, Oxford, before completing a History of Art M.Phil at Peterhouse College, Cambridge. Philip was diagnosed with HIV and Hep C in 2010, at the age of 24.

After five years of working as a lawyer in financial services, he left the City of London to pursue his activism full time in 2015. Coming to terms with his diagnoses has been an empowering process. He is associated with a number of charities, including Stonewall, the Terrence Higgins Trust, Positively UK, the Albert Kennedy Trust and Positive East.

There are a number of core components to Philip's activism,

including HIV awareness, co-infection with Hep C, and faith for LGBT (Lesbian, Gay, Bisexual & Transgender) people. In May he hosted an event on women and HIV in Parliament.

He recently organised a fringe event at the Conservative Party Conference on global LGBT rights.

He has columns in *Gay Times*, *The Huffington Post* and *Hep Magazine*. He contributed a chapter to a book called *The Power of My Faith*, discussing his journey with Christianity.

Christianity nourishes Philip's life, propelling him forwards. He is working on a semi-autobiographical book on stigma, called *Positive Damage*.

He is a happy, healthy, successful and POSITIVE man."

Employability

A Corporate Career & A Passion For Something Else...

I started my career in news/publishing at the age of 17 years old with my first 'career job' (I'll call it), working in sales for a local newspaper and my passion, love and career ambition grew from there. My career in corporate publishing continued to span over 15 years crossing over sales and marketing divisions until I climbed the steep ladder up to the highest possible level, despite it being a tremendously male-dominated industry. At the peak of my career I was working across Europe with over five hundred staff across several countries under my direction – and I loved every single second of it, the pressure, the achievement and pride but more so the people I worked with. I have always loved people.

I'm pretty traditional and old-fashioned at heart, I was raised in an ethical and hardworking family who, despite themselves not being particularly ambitious, supported me all the way through my career goals and I simply wouldn't be here without them.

Owning A Business Was Not Enough...

As I said, I've always been ambitious, so it made total sense to me in 2005 to launch my own company bringing my experience, skill and profession into focus in the route of a female owned marketing agency. It was always my goal to employ people, not a huge amount but enough to create the 'family' environment and stability I loved from my career days, so as soon as I could, I did. We now employ over twenty members of staff across the three offices and I couldn't be happier with my choice of 'team'.

Very early on in my company I volunteered on a local Government board which lobbied for employability and SME development nationally. As I said I love people, not only my own teams but externally I am passionate and enthusiastic about people generally and I care avidly that people from all walks of life deserve the very best support in order to achieve their own goals. Ten years on and I still sit on the same board and spend time on lobbying, policy representation and visiting Parliament in London. Here I raise the most prominent issues in employability across my region and the UK generally, bringing them to the attention of those at the top.

A statement I heard time and time again was 'the skills coming through the door don't match what we need as a company', this was echoed by not a few but literally hundreds of organisations I met across the country and across all sectors and provisions. It's not that I think there's a blame culture in this, it's neither the schools, colleges or job agencies fault. It's simply that there is a dramatic lack of clarification on curriculum, employability and training providers about what firms actually need in their recruitment journeys, and neither side is listening or acting.

The biggest concern (I believe) is that quite simply the unemployed, generally speaking are significantly and poorly represented when it comes to relevant and necessary employment skills. Employers shout about what they are looking for but providers are quite frankly restricted under red-tape to deliver the demands. I'm not simply speaking about young people just out of school I'm talking about the long-term unemployed, the difficult to reach individuals from dis-advantaged and unfortunate backgrounds. Whose education authorities, employment providers and indeed employers steer away from, because those are the people who will be the most challenging to recruit and place – but in my opinion and experience from my own recruitment processes, they will be your most loyal, hardworking and passionate employees!

Could I Do More To Help?

So, here my personal journey in employability and 'giving-back' started. Since 2009 I have made it my commitment to do what I can regionally to combat this issue, playing my part in plugging this gap and giving people the best chances of success, both within my own organisation and externally.

It all started when I approached local training providers and job agencies to ask them to send these 'difficult to place' individuals to me, for some voluntary work-experience. It took a while at first to convey the offering, for organisations to trust me as an employer and to understand the fact that I wasn't merely looking for 'free labour'.

No they don't get paid, but what they do get is experience within a working environment, coaching and one-to-one peer group mentoring which no one else offers anywhere in the UK.

In the past six years I as a business owner, and we as a company have helped over 260 individuals go into sustainable, relevant employment with a program I have personally led and developed, working in conjunction with providers such as the British Chamber of Commerce, Probation & Crime Commission Services, Job Centre, Derbyshire LEP, Sheffield City Region and Derbyshire County Council to create a non-profit program that supports local employment on a sustainable and direct impact level.

It's after the success of this program (*that I fully funded myself for six years*), that I decided helping 200 people locally simply wasn't enough – what if we could help double that? Or triple? In our minds, there should be a 'place' for anyone regardless of background, culture or academia to go and gain real valuable, employer-led support outside of the usual channels, so in 2015 we registered a non-profit Community Interest Company (CIC) called Brighter Futures Employability Derbyshire.

Why Do I Do It?

This is an easy one. I do it because I like people. I want the best for them, both professionally and personally. I was very lucky to have such a tremendous, exciting and rewarding career, because I worked hard and gave 100%. I'm not the brightest or best at what I do (there will always be someone better than you, I learnt that lesson a long time ago), but there will only ever be one best you. Everyone deserves that, we all deserve to be the best representation of what we can become, and everyone deserves the support, guidance and dedication to help them get there.

Whether your 'dream job' is to be a CEO of a multi-award-winning company, or a part-time commercial cleaner – is there a difference? I don't think so. If that's your dream then why shouldn't you go for it?

Both myself as the CEO/Chair and my brilliant team (*who all operate on a voluntary basis*), are incredibly passionate about our cause, we not only see the facts and figures at the end of each quarter, but we meet the people behind them, we see the direct impact that our program has on people's lives and it's not just about employment.

We have seen the shyest, most unemployable (on paper) individuals walk through our doors on day-one with their heads down, avoiding all eye-contact and achieving the lowest academic scores on our assessment papers. To go on to present to a room of professionals, increase literacy and maths skills, gain new found confidence and challenge their own family networks, and ultimately go on to achieve their self-created career goals. Gaining sustainable and rewarding work across a range of sectors from manufacturing, to office, retail and even within the public sector Police Force, GP (NHS) and high-technology creative industries – because of us, but also because of them, their self-belief and commitment to working through their own personal challenges to become the best person they can be.

Bumps In The Road...

The journey hasn't been without its challenges. Huge ones to be honest, which at times had me thinking *'shall I just give it up'* –

but it's not about me and the deflation I sometimes feel when we are turned down for a potential program. Boosting funding opportunity for the hundredth time, that could see us doing so much more; it's about the people we started this venture for: It's about the two-hundred and sixty individuals now in sustainable and happy employment, because of us. It's about the self-belief and skills we have developed in every single one of the people we have had through our doors, their self-confidence and life-changing environments, and it's about the wider impact it's had on our local region's employment figures.

How Much Does Our Program REALLY Help Our Community?

Working isn't just about income, it's about confidence, satisfaction, and self-value. It's about contributing to society in a meaningful way and making lasting connections with others. Helping people that face prejudice into work, means standing up to inequality and isolation. Sometimes life leads us down a dark road and we need a little help seeing the light... that is what our program does for people.

Let me share with you some recent employability analysis: as a region (where we are based), Derbyshire itself does have a small proportion of the population aged 16-64 that are claiming out-of-work benefits compared to England as a whole. But this is still an issue; just 1.1% people in Derbyshire are currently included on the claimant count; however, this is a lot less than last year in February 2015 and lower than the 1.8% claimant in England as a whole.

Although the unemployment stats have decreased there are still 6,155 people aged 16-64, which have claimed universal credit or job seekers allowance in Derbyshire alone in September 2016. 32.3% of all job seekers allowance claimants have been unemployed for a year or more.

This is why I feel that I need to do as much as I can to help those that want to get back into work. Most people do genuinely struggle to get into employment because they lack in employability skills, whereas some don't want to try to get a career. You can't label all the unemployed the same; individuals just need that extra help on a personal care level, we are not all sheep in a field.

In six years our program has helped over 260 unique individuals find themselves in stable employment, not just a job but something they love and can enjoy getting up to each morning.

98.9% of all individuals we have taken through our program have stayed in contact with us for the duration, with some people even referring family and friends to share their experience and improve lives for others they know.

In our experience, it's easy for real people, with complex lives and problems, to become just statistics and numbers (*i.e. numbers don't convey the struggles faced by many*).

There Are People Behind The Numbers...

Let's look at employment advice first of all – Through traditional routes, individuals seeking work and fitting within the 'long-term unemployed bracket' are given a label (e.g. unemployed, unskilled, disadvantaged, not fit for work, etc.) - now if you speak to these people, you'll find they often feel like another number in the statistics, but why should they?

Employers and providers should not passively accept the stereotypes associated with these individuals. People going through this difficult and stressful time of seeking employment (some may be in this position for no fault of their own, think about the hundreds over the last few years who have found themselves suddenly and tragically unemployed through company closures and redundancies – many on the job market for the first time in their lives) are individuals and to accept the subliminal messages from these labels is not only self-depreciating but also unproductive.

What Does The Programme We Run Look Like?

I made it my mission to not only create a program that works for the people coming through it (as in a customised, unrestricted approach), but also one that offers real end to end value for employers.

Our 'programme' is essentially developed around work-placement environments – so candidates (people), sign up for either an 8 or 12 week program. Again this is unpaid, in which time they receive a totally customised programme of development (CPD), which works towards building their 'dream' skills, characteristics and academia. That increases the chances of gaining the type of employment they are looking for, this traditionally includes:

1. Skills Assessments – we see where people are and the 'vision' of where they want to be
2. CPD – Building on their existing strengths and aligning weaknesses – what help is needed
3. Employability skills and soft skills – training and development in groups and 1-2-1
4. Personal development – looking at them as a person and working on a 1-2-1 level to provide on-hand guided mentoring and support – with an employer vision to make them the best they can possibly be and ultimately 'ready for work' in all senses
5. Work experience – A HUGE part of our program is getting them into the workplace. Teaching valuable work-ethic in a supportive environment for them to 'test and see' as well as gain real-life and valuable recent experience that they can then talk about to future employers
6. Continued growth – developing all the skills and lessons they have learnt and adapting that to a work environment and skills assessment, matching to the jobs they want
7. Job Application guidance and support from CV writing, covering letters right through to interview mocks and presentation skills – delivered by employers who actually interview people for jobs.
8. An employer's report – the final part of their program is their input into an accurate and representative report, which we create as a potential employer. Our honest feedback and opinion on them as an

individual, their characteristics, skills and what type of work they would thrive in for them to take away and share with perspective employers as a 'fact sheet' driven by an employer

Being proactive and making an effort during unpaid work WILL help you enter employment. For example, in addition to also achieving the tremendous numbers we do for people entering employment as a direct result to our intervention. We've also personally hired placements into permanent roles as a result of meeting them during our scheme.

My Advice To You…

First off, go for your goals. That's the most important one. Don't ever let ANYONE tell you, you can't do something, if your dream is to start your own company, amazing – equally, if it's to work within a small company, as an Office Administrator and get a great work/life balance, that too is amazing.

Sometimes you may find yourself in a situation you never thought you would be in, there is always a way to change the situation you are in. Always have faith in everything you do and if you believe in yourself anything is possible.

There are many organisations that can help you get back into employment whether it be the government or a private organisation, people are always there to help. You can find these by simply searching for charities or non- profit organisations online. If you don't have any internet access at home you can always go to a nearby library to use their computers, or even going into your local job centre to see how they can offer to help you. If none of those options are available to you for whatever reason, call or visit your local Citizens Advice Bureau or Council. Do not delay seeking help or information. Always accept any help that comes your way and remember these people or organisations want to help you to the best ability that they can.

Another piece of strong advice I'll give you is <u>be honest</u>. Acknowledge your situation (*even if it is difficult and upsetting*) and be truthful with yourself and those trying to help you. Deluding yourself about your situation, difficulty, and future prospects may be temporarily comforting, but leads to inactivity.

People all over the world overcome disadvantage by being proactive and seeking change, not simply accepting without challenging or challenging without thinking.

My Perspective As An Employer...

As a company we want the ***best*** people in our company. I don't just mean skills, for me the first thing I look for is personality and personal culture. Will you fit in with my existing team and how? As a company owner this is imperative to me as I need to know you will work as a collaborative team and fit within the existing skills and weaknesses (we all have them) we are building on.

I've learnt during my extensive career that recruitment is about the people. I have interviewed, assessed and recruited thousands of applicants over the years and took a select few into my teams to continue to develop and grow with the companies I've worked for. The skills can be taught but personality and company culture 'fit' can't, no matter how you sugar coat it.

As an employer, generally speaking 'we' look for the following things in a person:

- Attractiveness/ 'Realness of a CVs (both unpaid and paid work)
- Attitude & Positively – the 'real you' so they can see how you would fit in with them
- Personal presentation (what you 'look' like – thinking of the five senses)
- Soft Skills – basic literacy and maths, presentation skills, motivation, commitment, willingness to learn, ambition and team acumen
- Demonstrated skills/ experience – Not text-book but how you applied this in work/ life
- Disclosure – an open and reflective dialogue and honesty about your situation and a demonstration of commitment/ willingness for the chance to prove yourself

Why Is Our Program Different?

Ultimately I am an employer. Apart from it being my passion and something I love, I also have a successful thriving business to run (my marketing agency **Brighter Directions)** and I need staff to help the company move forward.

In the last five years, the majority of my recruitment has been driven through our non-profit activities. We have found the best people for the roles available through our work placement schemes, and as a business this has meant that my recruitment costs and resources have been reduced, yet I have not lost out on selecting the best people from our talent pools, it's a win, win situation!

What Other Help Is Out There?

Despite my comments earlier, there are still loads of resources out there to help people looking for work. Be it local provisions, such as Jobcentre's or tools like blogs, YouTube clips and advice on the website of how to get the best start – and, of course our personal programs run throughout Derbyshire (if you are lucky enough to live near us).

Widely speaking, unfortunately, what help is available can depend on personal situation, and the capacity and criteria of organisations. Some organisations might only offer help to people from a specific demographic group (e.g. young people, women, ex-offenders, etc.) or people in specific circumstances (e.g. unemployed for over 12 month). Some organisations' criteria can be arbitrary and not reflect the reality of people's disadvantage and need. This can be frustrating especially if you fall in an 'unpopular' or 'in-between' group.

The beauty about my employability program is that it's open to everyone. We are not restricted to your background, culture, situation or environment for skills. We specialise in working with the 'unpopular' or 'in-between' groups. BUT, there aren't local organisations in all disadvantaged communities, many of the one's that do have small capacity (i.e. *limited funds and resources, like us*). We rely on funding. At the moment we are limited to what we can deliver through my own money being invested in the company, which I will never get back. In the future like many charities and non-profits we need money to keep thriving, which is what we're working on currently through external and public bodied routes to funding.

Finding available help can be difficult. Here are some solutions:

- Approach government services (job centers, councils, advice bureau). This will differ depending on area but there is usually someone who will be able to point you in the right direction.
- Try to search online for organisations like BF (note that many small charities and not for profits are not well advertised). If you don't have access to the internet, or have a disability that makes it difficult to see or read, visit your local library and ask for help or ask a friend/relative (if possible).
- Work placements and unpaid work. Talk to organisations (for example Job Centre) that send people to mandatory placements. You could also contact local employers directly to ask them if they take on work placements.

Even if it's not necessarily a job/place you want to be in, <u>think positively</u> about it. Even if attendance is not voluntary, there are hidden opportunities so take advantage. For example, new skills, job references, chance to make friends/contacts, escape isolation, possible paid employment.

What's Next For Us?

Brighter Futures Employability Derbyshire is still on our journey to make the world a better place, in terms of future employability anyway. As a business woman and a community leader, my feelings towards employability in the UK is that we need to create an employer-led solution. One that supports Government initiatives to bring down unemployment rates nationally, but it can't be done in isolation.

Sure, we're doing an amazing job in our region but we shouldn't be the only ones. It's taken us blood, sweat, toil and many tears to get to where we are, and we're still fighting to do more. What we need is funding in the future to enable us to run this program bigger and wider than we are currently doing. For people to join us on our vision of helping everyone gain accessible and relevant work employability across the UK. Our dream is big and we won't give up!

Claire Curzon

About The Author

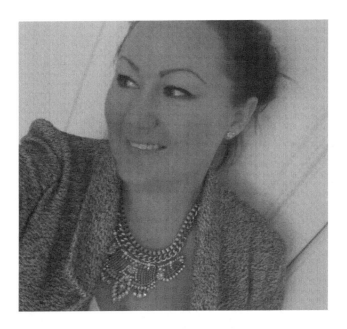

Claire Curzon is a successful female business leader in the world of marketing. After leaving the safe corporate world of marketing to launch her own agency multi-award-winning marketing agency, **Brighter Directions** eleven years ago, she now stands at the forefront of a male-dominated industry. Claire has built her reputation around strong ethics, quality provision and her team around her, providing leadership, support and motivational demonstration of quality, leading by example.

People have always been central to her passion, throughout her career. As a result while growing her own business she also launched and funded a regional non-profit charity that supports her local community and economy by providing tangible and effective commercial led support to people seeking sustainable employment, particularly the 'difficult to reach' communities who find employment prospects most difficult to achieve. Her mission, to create an employer led program which not only addresses the skills gap nationally, reduces unemployment figures and contributes to the economy, but one that is also focused around the people directly through soft skills, employability skills and personal development.

Everyone deserves a job they love....

Should you wish to contact Claire or find out more, visit her:

Website: www.brighterdirections.co.uk

Twitter: www.twitter.com/brighter

Website: www.employabilityderbyshire.org.uk

You Will Amount To Nothing In Life

Whenever anyone asks me how life is, I have a standard response now. I am not living my dream because I would never have allowed myself to believe that life could be this good. Life is better than my wildest dream. Now I'm aware that sounds like an exaggeration but I promise you it is true.

I currently live on the Mid North coast of New South Wales, Australia. Today has been a typical day for me at this stage of my life. I began the day at a leisurely pace, gradually easing into some business development work. As with most days, I'm at home. This was followed by a walk on the beach, holding hands with my wife. Our local beach is simply stunning and stretches from horizon to horizon. It's not unusual to see dolphins playing in the ocean and eagles soaring above. Quite regularly there will be a mere handful of people there and some days you can have the beach all to yourself. Today as we walked on the beach we talked about the year that is closing and the year ahead. This year has been astonishingly positive, not least in visiting four countries I've never been to before. Next year I already have four overseas trips booked and expect that to increase.

But let me introduce myself before going any further. My name is Alex Couley. At the point of writing I'm fifty six years old. I was born and lived most of my life in England. My wife and I migrated to Australia fourteen years ago. That was when the real magic in life began. It was in that move that we discovered our personal secret to happiness.

I discovered relatively late in life that I had been given lessons throughout my life that had always been pointing me in the direction that I needed to go. In my infinite wisdom I had ignored the same glaring messages time and time again. Therefore my intention in sharing my story is to share what I have learnt with you. I hope that in doing so some of you will benefit. As I have already mentioned the learning finally came home to roost when we migrated to Australia.

However in order to make sense of that part of the journey I will need to share with you a bit more background. I will also need to describe how the same teaching arose in different forms and at significant intervals across my life span until I realised my truth.

Let's begin with a brief description of my childhood and the two major challenges I faced. I was born and spent my childhood in Newcastle-Upon-Tyne - an industrial city in the North East of England. It would be easy to say that we were poor and that life was tough but to be honest that's just hindsight. At the time it didn't feel like that. We were living life like most people around us. I think that poor is a relative concept, if everyone you interact with has the same standard of living, it just feels normal. And it did. I grew up in a very loving family home. Despite the lack of material possessions I knew that my parents loved me and my two sisters. My parents both worked hard but the economic situation was very difficult. They never complained and only later did I realise the sacrifices they had made for the children.

My first big challenge in life was my health. I was born with a cardiac problem. One of the main valves in my heart was narrowing and my life was at risk. The medical staff advised my parents that it would be best to wait until I was at least thirteen to conduct the necessary surgery to correct the issue. That way my heart would have grown sufficiently to increase the chances of a positive outcome. Unfortunately when I reached the age of eight it became apparent that I wasn't going to make it that long.

The plan was brought forward and I underwent open heart surgery. The operation they performed on me is relatively straight forward now but at the time was not routine in children. Reflecting from today's perspective, it wasn't exactly keyhole surgery and I was left with a very substantial scar.

Clearly I didn't know this then but I now know that giving consent for this risky procedure was very tough on my parents. The operation went well but I had to be treated in a hospital a long way from my family home. Visiting me was a big commitment for my family. We didn't have a car and it was a long journey on public transport. My sisters, naturally, were also in need of my parent's time, so one parent visited me whilst another took care of the home.

After a period of convalescence in hospital I was finally discharged. Again, unknown to me at the time, my parents were told that if I made it to eighteen I would lead a full life but that reaching eighteen was not guaranteed. My most vivid childhood memories are not of playing in the park or similar but of long treks to see a cardiologist. Due to the lengthy hospitalisation and subsequent convalescence I missed a lot of schooling. When I did go back to school I was given a note to carry with me at all times. It told the teachers of my heart troubles and excused me from physically exerting activities.

The focus became my health. Everyone meant well, but to me it felt like I was very different from my peers. The scar didn't help. Over the years my visits to the cardiologist became less frequent, gradually reducing to annually. They continued until I was eighteen at which point I was given the all-clear.

Being a child I didn't know that our brain has been designed to seek out evidence to support whatever you tell it is true. I will build on this later but for now, suffice to say, that with everyone telling me I was ill, all I saw was evidence to prove that this was indeed true. I learnt to believe that I was not capable of things because of my supposed ill health. Whereas in reality people endure much worse and flourish.

On that note let us jump to the next childhood challenge. This time it wasn't an individual one but universal to all my peers. The area of Newcastle where we grew up was heavily dependent upon shipbuilding for employment. Unfortunately for our generation as we approached school leaving age the shipbuilding industry went into heavy decline.

Everyone's expectation for us was very low. I can best illustrate this through one event I recall as if it were yesterday. When I was fourteen years old without warning our teacher stopped the class. She said that there was no point in any of us continuing to study because we wouldn't amount to anything in life. She continued, saying that half of us would be unemployed for life and the other half would spend the majority of our time in prison. Looking back, the most shocking thing was that neither I nor my fellow students were surprised by this. When I said earlier that everyone had low expectations for us, that included ourselves.

Not long before I left school my uncle said to me that I would look back on these as the best days of my life. I remember being horrified by that thought. Thankfully he was completely wrong. I left school at sixteen with no educational qualifications. I left school on Friday and registered for unemployment benefit on the following Monday, truly believing that the teacher was right.

Remember what I said earlier about the brain seeks evidence to support what is told is true? Well there is another dimension to that. In order to keep us safe our brain has evolved to have what's known as the negativity bias. That means we are hardwired to remember negative information longer and more vividly than positive information. The teacher mentioned above had unintentionally activated this process in me. This was to the extent that, when I recently spoke at Harvard University, I still hear her voice saying you will amount to nothing. Again we will return to this but you cannot overestimate the power of the negativity bias and the need to challenge it.

By this time in life I was already being shown the lesson that has become the foundation of the most recent decade. Unfortunately I wasn't able to see it. My spell of unemployment was just short of one year. Bearing in mind that by that stage I was still only seventeen, I had given up all hope of a positive future. I couldn't make sense of why life had to be this way. As luck would have it I was fortunate to get a few temporary positions in roles I didn't enjoy but at least gave me some sense of dignity.

Then from nowhere came the first major positive event I can recall. I applied for and was accepted into a mental health nurse training programme. I wasn't to know this at the time but that move set my life up to be one of serving others and led ultimately to finding my true purpose.

I'm going to give you a brief overview of the next two decades. Clearly in any person's life twenty years is a long time and includes many events. There were some very significant moments but I want to get us to the point of migrating to Australia. So forgive me for rushing through this section of my life.

After three years of study, I went to qualify as a mental health nurse. Up until that point the hospital had recruited nearly all the staff it trained. Unfortunately the year I qualified the economy was dipping even further and the majority of us received two letters. One saying you've qualified and the other saying you no longer have a job. Deja vu, just like when I left school.

At the same time I had met the woman who was to become my first wife. We married and moved to Cambridge in the south east of England, where we were both employed in a large hospital as psychiatric nurses. The years in Cambridge were to shape the rest of my life in the mental health field. I grew rapidly in my skill set and was promoted very quickly. Alongside this, our family grew too with the birth of three children. I won't talk about my children beyond this point. But I want to share with you that I am very proud of all three of them. They each have blossomed into very different adults. Carving their own paths out in life. Wherever life takes them I know they will do well.

After nine years in Cambridge work opportunities brought our family back to the north east. I managed a mental health facility in Northumberland. During this period of my life my first marriage came to an end. The children stayed with their mother and I moved out to live on my own.

Then my life took an unexpected turn when I met the person who eventually became my second wife. For the first time in my life, I felt like I was in the company of someone who believed in me and encouraged me to be the best version of myself. As you will see later we have gone on to craft a life of true happiness together.

I said I would move through these decades quickly and so I will. One day I had a very bad day at work. One of those days where you say I don't want to be here anymore. On a whim I decided I would migrate to Australia. I had never been there and knew very little about the country beyond what I had seen on TV. I was interviewed in London and the interviewer said when you get there you will live like a lottery winner. I had no idea how true that would become.

From that point it wasn't as plain sailing as I had anticipated. My childhood cardiac challenges came back to haunt me. In the medical for migration they found I had very high blood pressure. The Australian authorities wouldn't allow me to travel there until this was rectified. The resulting medication experimentation, trying to find a solution, only served to push the blood pressure up further. Months went by trying to resolve the blood pressure issue. The negativity bias I mentioned earlier kicked in at this point. I came very close to giving up but my wife kept me strong. Then one day the visa arrived. I thought I was going to be given a four year visa but had been granted permanent residency in Australia. Superb news.

In January 2003 I moved to Australia with my wife. We left the north east of England in the heart of Winter. It was minus six degrees Celsius at its warmest. We arrived into Melbourne in the middle of the night. It was thirty four Celsius. My immediate thought was, how can human beings live in this? In understanding my story I need to share with you that at this point I promised my wife that I wouldn't attempt to build a career. I would sit back, perform a junior role and cruise through until retirement. How wrong can someone be?

Early into my time in Australia emerged another key figure. The second person to really believe in me. I attended some training that was meant to improve my skills at work. One of the people teaching the course became a dear friend but more importantly an inspiring mentor. As said the intention behind the training was to increase my skill set but in fact it became a blue print by which I've lived life ever since.

So here is the core of what I was taught; Most people travel through life focusing on what society says is success. They aspire towards the bigger house, more money, promotion etc. Particularly in western nations we are taught that success is defined by achieving your goals and sometimes it is ok for that to be at the expense of others.

But there is another way and it leads to a greater level of perceived happiness. First you begin by working out what your values are. Now that sounds easy but it's not. What really matters to you, is not a question we often take time to reflect upon. Once you are there your life should be constructed around striving to have more of these values in your everyday experience. Also key to this process is understanding that human beings evolved to become the cooperative species. We were never the fastest animal on the African savannahs, we didn't have the biggest teeth or claws, we became the dominant species by learning to cooperate with one another. This is now hard wired into us.

Therefore it's not just about your goals, it's about striving towards your core values to be of service to all of those you encounter. Then to add to all of this, the process is far more successful if you are moving towards something you want more of, rather than away from something you don't. These are distinctly different motivations that cause different outcomes for people. Like most people I've encountered I was taught the opposite. Avoid the negative, rather than strive with purpose towards what can be.

There is one more major component to this process that I will share with you before we come to the end of my story (or at least my story so far).

Most of what is described above is popularised in sayings like "follow your bliss', follow your passion or dreams". These pieces of advice are very often dismissed as fanciful and promising the impossible. I would argue that if you are exposed to the science behind this, are taught how to do it and crucially work at it, then it can be utterly life transforming. It was for me.

So let's look at how my life did transform by integrating these concepts. Despite my promise to my wife I was rapidly promoted at work. I began to teach my clients and colleagues these principles and saw dramatic results. The more I saw changes in others the more I integrated it into my own life. On a very personal note one shining moment was becoming an Australian citizen. I have to tell you, at the citizenship ceremony they played Scotland the brave, to this day I am confused by that. I'd expected something like waltzing Matilda. Anyway back to the story. Despite the successes, I still had my own limiting beliefs. I tried to stay positive but it was hard.

That teacher from the past still haunted me saying "you won't amount to much". I told you earlier that the trainer became a friend and mentor. Over dinner, one day, he challenged my self-limiting beliefs and encouraged me to explore new horizons. He taught me to stop focusing on what I believed I couldn't do and put my attention on what excited me even if I thought it wasn't possible. That conversation directly led to a major career change. I went on to study coaching. Amazingly I was excited and invigorated by life in a way that I had never thought was possible. At that stage what I didn't know was that there was even better to come.

Like most professions there is a lot of nonsense written about coaching. It is simply about helping people to become the best version of themselves given their personal circumstances. Of course there are skills involved in doing this and the best coaches have learnt to be very good at what they do. I believe however that anyone can learn these skills.

I found that everything I had learnt in the mental health field translated beautifully into this new arena. Despite this I kept on working in the mental health sector thinking that I could never become a professional coach. Over time as I watched others coach, people who were making a decent living at it, I began to soften my view but still thought I didn't have the experience of running a business. I'd only ever been an employee. I sought the advice of other professional coaches, most discouraged me, just like in my childhood with my health and my teacher with life prospects, they focused on the negative. They told me of all of the things that could go wrong and why it was too risky.

Then into my life walked the third person to believe in me. A lecturer on the course I was completing did the exact opposite to the others. This young woman again challenged my self-limiting beliefs. She, yet again, pushed me to focus on what could be rather than paying attention to all of the barriers.

Soon after I set up my own business and it boomed. Despite being told by "experts" I would struggle to find enough work exactly the reverse happened. I simply couldn't believe how easy it felt and most importantly how happy I was. I established a business built around the idea of my definition of coaching, helping others to be the best version of themselves. The business flourished. I contacted the lecturer mentioned above and asked to meet her for coffee. The plan was to say thank you for believing in me when others didn't. That wasn't what happened. When we met for coffee we fed off each other's desire to make a difference in the world and we agreed to set up another business in partnership.

Now I found myself running one business and jointly running another. I still had no formal training in how to develop or manage a business and to this day haven't. I worked on the basis of not focusing on making money but focusing on giving the best value I possibly could. This approach has never let me down.

Shortly after setting the joint business up, myself and my business partner went on to coauthor a book on coaching. We developed and published our unique model of coaching. I've now published numerous times, presented at many conferences, trained hundreds of people and never struggled for business. I'm not going to write this and pretend it's all been easy, there have been many moments of doubt. To become very successful you do have to take risks - and I have. That said the risks have been what has made the journey fun. I haven't mentioned that word, fun, so far but I would like to stress that whatever you choose to strive for, make sure you are having fun on the way. If it all comes to an end you can always say at least I had a ball whilst it lasted.

In a moment I am going to take us back to this year but I want to take you on one slight diversion first. A few years ago now, I was asked to speak at Harvard about why I am involved in the coaching world. I was among a group of people talking about the same subject. Most got up and did a sales pitch for their business. I chose to tell the story of the teacher who told me and my classmates that we wouldn't amount to anything. I said I wanted to be the voice that challenged the limiting stories others had been told. After I spoke a woman from New York approached me and said thank you for reminding everyone that not all of us come from privileged backgrounds.

The reason I share this with you is that I decided to stop telling the story of my childhood, thinking that the story itself limited me. I was wrong, the story isn't the issue. In fact your story is all you have. The secret is to own the story rather than let the story own you. In doing so you have the opportunity to reach out and inspire others. So my advice to you reader is share your story, no matter what it is, with pride.

Now back to where we began. This year started with a trip to the Canadian Rockies. It was a dream holiday. I had yearned for this trip from the age of fourteen but this year I did it in style. I flew to Canada business class and stayed in the top hotels throughout the Rockies. It was magnificent.

Business boomed and that has led me to deliver leadership development work to a number of multi-national companies. Mid-year saw me working in China, India and Thailand. Due to this success, my wife was able to leave work to travel with me. This sent our quality of life soaring. Remember I told you earlier that when I was interviewed to work in Australia, the interviewer said you will live like a lottery winner. Well I am not a multimillionaire but if I was I wouldn't change a single thing in my life. I live a life of abundance. So in that sense the person was absolutely correct.

I said earlier that there was one other major component to what changed my life, well here it is. When I needed it most there were people who came into my life who believed in me even when I didn't. They were the cheerleaders of my life, the people who walked alongside me when it seemed tough, the people who were brave enough to challenge my excuses head on and most of all the people who role modelled every word they uttered.

Of these people, special note has to go to my wife. She has been the greatest supporter of my journey, without her I'm sure I wouldn't have made it. I am eternally grateful for her love and belief in me. I would not be serving you well if I didn't share with you that part of the support from my wife has been the acceptance of the risks. Her standard response has always been to believe in me. I was always dismissive of terms like soul mate but in her I have truly found mine.

The negative voices deserve a mention too. They are not without merit. Each of them have contributed to who I am now and if I had the power I wouldn't change those voices either. There is an often used phrase, everyone who comes into your life brings a lesson. I think that is true but only if you consciously choose to make it so.

My closing comments to you are that "If I Can, You Can" is more than just a title for a book. It holds a core truth. It is possible, you'll need to focus upon what really matters to you and strive to have more of those things in your day to day life. You will also need to ignore those negative voices around you and find your team of people who believe in you. I promise you that they are there and they will keep you strong when it matters most. Of course none of this comes without work and an element of courage but the results are far better than you can imagine.

Finally I end with a request. If you encounter someone who is questioning whether or not they can achieve their dreams, no matter what their current circumstances, be the person who raises them up. Don't be the doubter; there are enough of them anyway. If you can find it in your heart to be the one who shares hope, it will raise your spirit too. Be the hope carrier you would like to meet.

Alex Couley

About The Author

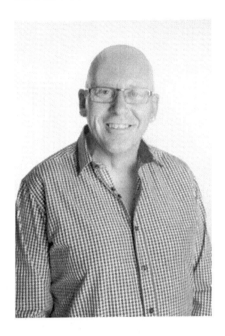

Alex Couley is recognised as an international figure in leadership development, coaching and positive psychology. He is a Director of the International Centre for Leadership Coaching, Director of ARC Consultancy and Leadership Programme Director at EduInfluencers. He is passionate about helping people achieve their personal best in any given situation and role modelling the same.

Sharing a post from my Facebook Page
the day I began to write this chapter:

"I met Alex Couley on the 5 February 2010 and he gently challenged me to question my perspective through compassion and authentic leadership; which has given me the drive to continue to pursue opportunities today that influence attitudes towards mental health and recovery. If you are pursuing professional development skills Alex Couley will bring the necessary integrity and expertise to empower yourself to effect positive change for yourself!"

If you'd like to find out more about Alex visit his:

Website: www.iclc.com.au

or Email: alex.couley@hushmail.com

Facebook: https://www.facebook.com/icleadershipcoaching/

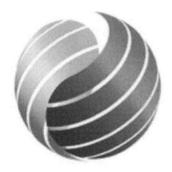

International Centre for
**LEADERSHIP
COACHING**

TOUCH

"What Consumes Your Mind, Controls Your Life"

Your thoughts and obsessions will determine how your life plays out and whether or not you are successful in what you hope to achieve. Anything that consumes your mind will control your life, and this will happen on both a conscious and a subconscious level. Your subconscious will work very hard to make what you believe will happen - actually happen - whether your expectations are positive or negative. When something consumes your mind it is hard to stop thinking about it, and this will take control of every aspect of your life.

Many people are self-destructive without even realising it, because they are consumed by negative thoughts. These thoughts are repeated so much that they can become a self-fulfilling prophecy. The same is also true with positive thoughts. Take a hard look at what consumes your thoughts and decide whether this is something that you want to have control of in your life. It is possible to change negative thought patterns and obsessions so that you have a better life, but only if you are willing to let go of any negative obsessions and redirect your thoughts in a more positive manner. Remember that what you think and believe can be changed when you get both your conscious and subconscious mind on board with the changes.

"What consumes your mind, controls your life." What you decide to obsess over in your mind... reviewing ... rewinding ... will ultimately be what controls you. It will be the CENTRE SCREEN of your life. And unless you change your mind, and change the channels, you will continue to see the frustrating flicker of that thing, that face, that obsession because you can't seem to move past whatever it is that has a hold on you. You feel your energy being depleted and your time being sucked away. If you can take a step back and look – truly LOOK – at the energy that this THING is taking from your life, you are ready to be honest.

Holistic healing is an approach to health and wellness that takes into consideration the whole person, addressing their physical, mental, and emotional health, and well-being, spiritual values, social lifestyle, and interaction with the environment. Holistic health is based on the natural principle that the whole is comprised of inter-reliant parts, and that when one part is not functioning at optimum levels, it impacts all of the other parts.

"TOUCH" focuses on all aspects of a person, not just the physical portion where ailments are most obvious. Physical symptoms can be alleviated by taking medication, but unless the whole person is treated, the actual root of the problem still exists. Holistic healing goes beyond merely treating symptoms, and instead uses them as a guide to address the root cause of the problem.

As an ongoing process and approach to life rather than just focusing on individual issues, "TOUCH" involves us in every aspect of the mind, body and soul relationship. With an objective of achieving optimum health and wellness, a holistic healer leads us on a journey of self-discovery and engages us in taking an active role and responsibility with regards to everyday choices.

The Core Arena's In Which I Treat Are:
Mind, Cells, Energy, Diet, Nutrition and Lifestyle. These are just some of the tools I will utilize to not only to help and support you

along your path to wellness, but most importantly, I will also endeavour to teach you as much as I can so that you can be proactive as well as empowered within the experience.

Cells

The cells in our bodies are continually being replaced and are developed from what currently exists in the body, it is essential that we become aware of the effects of our choices. Unhealthy foods, harmful substances, a toxic environment, and negative attitudes can result in flawed or damaged cells, resulting in healthy cells being replaced with sickly cells and ultimately leading to illness. Seemingly insignificant choices made each day accumulate in the mind and body, establishing our quality of life now and in the future. The focus and goal of holistic healing is to achieve the highest overall level of health and wellbeing through thoughtfully considered choices. While setbacks may occur, they are short-lived and the general flow is continually toward wellness.

Embracing holistic health and healing enables us to obtain wholeness within ourselves, which then naturally expands into increasing compassion and acceptance of others along with caring for our relationships and physical surroundings.

Every Cell in Your Body has a "Clock" in it. There is a natural healing force within you. It is your most powerful weapon against disease. Your body is a miracle of nature and has an extraordinary talent to heal itself. There is a powerful energy that can be transmitted through my hands to influence cells, cure disease and relieve pain.

Chakras

A network called the chakra system. In terms of medical intuition, these are our emotional centres, which link with our physical anatomy. Emotions are wired between the brain and the body. Each centre has a life situation and an emotion that affects an area of the body. This is the map that's going to help you create health.

Your body has an energy field. This energy field is called your "Aura". Sometimes due to trauma we experience "Negative Energy". Negative energy creates blockages and stops your natural healing ability.

Energy flows through your body along lines called meridians. When you are healthy this energy flows easily. If your energy flow is blocked then you may become unwell. Spiritual healing removes blockages along your energy paths. Once these blockages are removed your energy starts to circulate freely and you feel renewed.

We can have energy patterns stored from events that happened yesterday as well as from many years ago. Some of these patterns will be happy memories and others will be unpleasant or painful memories of something that happened to us. Sometimes we stash them away deep into some recess in our chakras and in our auras (the energy field around us). We try to forget about painful memories, but they don't really go away. Disease is a manifestation of unbalanced Energy. Healing is a way of balancing Energy.

Holistic

My approach as a holistic therapist is to help you understand how to nourish your body and spirit whilst you strive for inner harmony. I offer my clients support with no judgement. We share a proactive relationship which is employed to empower you along your path. This requires you live in accordance to nature, seasonal eating and listening to your body's needs.

Over the last 20 years of being a Holistic therapist I have seen a vast array of people from different walks of life with differing histories, values, beliefs and circumstances. The one overwhelming realization I have from listening to all their stories is that we are all the same. We all want the same things: To love and be loved, To belong, To be valued, To feel accepted, To be free, To feel connected, To be heard, To trust, To feel safe, To feel joy, peace, calm, To be true to ourselves, To know and live our purpose. And the root negative emotion that holds people back from fulfilling these needs? Fear.

Fear that we are not enough, good enough, smart enough, confident enough, thin enough, good looking enough, fast enough and that list goes on and on.

Self-healing always starts by removing negative energy blocks. Doctor's looks at your body, diagnose a problem and give you medicine. They don't always take into account your emotional and spiritual state. Your emotions can't be seen but play a huge factor in self-healing.

Stress and worry will eventually affect your body, so spiritual healing takes your emotions into account. The reason you are sick today is probably because of a build-up of negative emotions. The effects of worry and stress may not show up today but at some point they may show up as an illness. You won't know this and may look for other causes, which can lead you to taking medicines you don't need. All medicines have side effects.

Natural healing identifies the underlying source of your illness. Modern medicine deals with symptoms, natural healing understands causes. Negative energy is present in 99% of people living in modern society.

Remember, healing starts by removing negative energy blocks along your body's meridians. If you don't do this first, everything else, medicine, exercise and therapy will be diluted. Remember disease is when your body is out of balance.

"TOUCH THERAPY" is a Healing Journey. I never say "cure", or "do this and presto, you'll be cured." Healing is a process, a holistic process. And the word 'journey' indicates that it takes time, effort, and like any journey, there are twists and turns in the road, there are setbacks and calamities. But you press on and eventually you reach your destination. So how can you heal yourself and restore balance to your body, mind and soul, read Rachel's Story and her Journey to Wellness.

Rachel's Story

Rachel has suffered with eczema for most of her life with various severe episodes triggered by life experiences, her eczema comes and goes but at times of high stress it flares up significantly.

During the year of 2014 she developed eczema quite badly especially on her hands and face, giving a serious knock to her self-confidence and personal wellbeing. Rachel is a sensitive soul and because of this a vicious circle was created where the eczema would make her feel worse and she felt worse because the eczema had flared up – the worst kind of chicken and egg scenario.

She had moments of feeling her skin crawl and just wanted to rip the skin off because of the itching. It drove her to distraction; it affected her sleep, her job, her personal life, and became the defining negative element in her life. It was truly awful at times, and led Rachel to start to feel incredibly low.

She started to feel she had nowhere to turn, that people didn't understand her, and that she wanted to withdraw. Rachel felt she was in a transitional stage of life and knew that her eczema flared up when she felt stressed and angry, but she struggled to control those emotions and it meant that she had times when her eczema even stopped her from going outdoors. This was when Rachel reached rock bottom.

It was during an earlier point Rachel – a time when she had been subjected to high stress levels – that in 2010 she realised her emotional state was reflecting what happened to her eczema. She went through a very sad and demoralising situation and shortly thereafter the first little spot showed up. She realised this was the link to her eczema but she had no idea how to change this or where to seek help.

Rachel's childhood was spent watching her mothers' work as an artist. Like many little girls, Mum was a hero to Rachel, and as she grew older and the maternal bond grew stronger Rachel sought after her mother's acceptance, and respect as well as affection. Affection is a given from a parent, acceptance and respect is harder won. She naturally wanted to follow in her mother's footsteps – she developed her own interests in colour and drawings, and wanted to impress mum all the time.

The issue was that Rachel never quite had the natural flare and talent – people in the art world call this "The Art Eye" – you either had it or you didn't. Rachel's mother had this in bucket loads and her artwork was natural and effortless. Rachel had to try harder, much harder, due to her lack of natural talent and often felt knocked by her mother's well-meant critiques of her work.

These knocks were really felt as Rachel was so desperate to prove herself as an only child. Through her teenage years she became anxious, jealous, and at times angry with her mother, as she fought her emotions and tried to gain her acceptance.

All she wanted was her mum to say "well done, this is great, I'm proud of you" – sadly for Rachel these words never came. Her mother was a direct, hard-working, northerner, who offered praise lightly, and a scolding liberally. She believed the best medicine for Rachel was tough love – Rachel really wanted nurturing, and yearned for her mother to be softer, warmer. It led to some predictable clashes as she grew into a young woman – and at times they grew apart.

Rachel's mother was a very talented artist who was very successful financially and Rachel always pushed herself to be as good. The expectations Rachel put on herself were immense. She wanted her mother to be so proud of her. Rachel worked extremely hard to get good grades but art never came as naturally as it did for her mother. She spent many hours painting and trying to make a successful living, which consumed all of her time day and night. It took over her life, and the hours she had to put in just to make sure ends meet were a drain on her energy as the shadow of mums big house and shiny new cars were a constant reminder of how good her mother was and Rachel's relative lack of success.

Back to 2010 – the high stress moment was the passing of Rachel's mother from a quick illness. Rachel was distraught – despite the challenging nature of their relationship the loss of her mother before she felt she had fully been given her blessing wore heavily on Rachel's heart. She felt such loss and sadness in her soul.

This is a truly natural reaction to the loss of a loved one, but for Rachel, she had lost not only a parent but an idol. She felt no longer the urges to pursue her art – the acceptance she yearned for was never going to come now - the creative juices she used to have stopped flowing. She was sinking deeper and deeper into a darker place and a part of her was missing. Being an artist she couldn't feel the brush in her hand anymore. She was going through the motions, she eventually gave up painting and gave up her zest of life overall too – she questioned why she was alive.

Rachel's eczema over time became worse and was told she would need to go on steroids in a somewhat matter-of-fact routine way. She had been on and off steroids for years and at times when it was at its worse she could not sleep at night. She had always wondered how long she would have to stay on steroids and had to apply aqueous cream, she saw no results. Doctors, pills, creams, nothing worked. Armed with her prescription, she felt as if she didn't have the correct tools for her fight, she felt low and thought – "this is me now". Rachel searched for an alternative and found me on the internet. She was desperate, a final throw of the dice, she made an appointment for her first visit.

Touch Therapy

Skin covers our entire body, every thought we think and every word we say and every intention we ever have passes through our skin on its way to communicate with the outside world. So it doesn't just protect us from the world, quite the opposite is true, it translates our inner being to the surface.

It is constantly in contact with and intimate with our inner workings. Because of this, skin reflects how we feel about ourselves. Skin forms our barrier, our identity. It forms what we perceive as 'us' and delineates us from the rest of the world. Skin is our outer projection of our inner truths. In short, skin is our boundary.

Skin can speak to us through the location of eczema patches, acne, dry tight skin, hives, changes in hair growth, pigmentation, wrinkles, stretch marks and more.

Skin can speak subtly through chronic messages that it whispers to you your entire life. Or skin can scream loudly and angrily during acute transitions and times of crisis. But no matter how your skin speaks to you, there is always a message to be appreciated.

Hearing that message and honouring what boundary issue is going on in your life, taking steps to shore up or relax your boundaries as need be, adjusting them to better support your inner spirit, often this supports your skin issue on a deeper level then any ointment, cream, lotion or cleanser will ever be able to.

Eczema is a result of high stress levels and toxins. Its side effects include a poor functioning liver, and a week immune system. Weak liver function plays a significant role because the liver is largest cleansing organ in the body. Therefore, if the liver is not cleansing the body correctly or enough, the unfiltered toxins must then be released from the skin, the largest organ in our bodies. Lastly, a delicate immune system is powerless against allergens and cannot fend the body from skin irritants.

The skin represents how we present ourselves to the world, as a reflection of how we see ourselves. It is highly sensitive and absorbent so it reflects minor changes in our internal and external environment. When we show healthy, glowing skin to the world, we feel good about ourselves, complete in our own reflection. When our skin is irritated or inflamed, it is an indication that there is a frustration stemming from how we see ourselves.

Any consistent imperfection of the skin is a sign that we are seeing ourselves as inadequate in some way, an imperfect self-perception will naturally create an imperfect exterior.

You feel as though whatever you do is not good enough so you see yourself as imperfect or not as you would prefer to be. This causes you to be hard on yourself, and everything that you do. This creates tension and frustration. This frustration is simply repressed energy that could be better used to focus on your good qualities rather than your shortfalls. You need to learn to love and accept yourself, knowing that everything that you are and do is as it is meant to be. This will alleviate your frustration and allow you to use your energy to create with the freedom of self-expression.

I looked at the location of the eczema as this is a key telling point - e.g. behind an ear if you dislike people gossiping about you, on an arm if you feel held back, or on your back if you think people are talking about you behind your back.

Rachel tended to absorb criticism instead of asserting herself. She was very prone to making 'rash' decisions and judgements and putting herself down by focusing on her flaws and not celebrating the beauty of life.

Why are you so uncomfortable in your skin? Expression in skin cells. The direct result of losing someone or something you love is profound grief. And that hollow, meaningless feeling that accompanies loss does not lead to art. Yet we know art is the answer. Rachel's life story seemed to be influenced in many areas of her life with self-sabotaging beliefs and holding on to and not being able to release these. Rachel had been putting off using her hands and in turn using her creative ability.

When Rachel visited me for the first time she knew subconsciously it was time for an inner/outer detox. Your eczema is a message that change is sorely needed. When you accept that your body is your friend, not an enemy, ultimate healing becomes possible.

If Rachel wanted the eczema to go away, she had to get to the emotional cause, and release the fears and sadness. To express such feelings of fear and insecurity. She was bottling things up, eczema was her body's desperate attempt to say that she was scared. There was a tension, which cannot be described as anger, more as frustration. It seemed she couldn't find her voice.

A stressful lifestyle can affect the intestine greatly. When one is faced with emotional or psychological stress on a daily basis, the body produces cortisol (a hormone) which affects the intestinal tract by destroying friendly bacteria. The digestive system becomes impaired. A chain reaction can lead to a whole host of diseases including that of eczema.

Rather than dividing illness into "emotional" or "psychosomatic" and "physical," I see emotions as one factor in all skin diseases. Some skin problems are like the common experience of blushing: an emotional event produces a direct and dramatic change in the skin. Emotional stress may be the sole cause of a few symptoms, but is more typically a trigger of the flare-ups of an ongoing medical condition.

Eczema sufferers are able to identify specific emotional triggers. People who seek medical attention for a skin problem experience significant underlying psychological turmoil. This is critically important because emotional problems can keep even the most sophisticated medical treatment from working, which unfortunately is a steroid that suppresses your immune response and thins your skin over time. When you are more methodical and holistic about your treatment, your skin, body and spirit has no choice but to balance itself.

The three primary ways that toxins enter the blood stream and thus the body are: through the digestive system (eaten), through the respiratory system (breathed in), and through the skin (absorbed).

"Touch Therapy Journey"

Touch Therapy took Rachel on a new journey, as I gradually started heal her and introduce more of a creative lifestyle with plenty of opportunity for self-expression. Here's how I treated the problem of eczema....

Chakra Healing In Each Session

I started by removing energy blocks. When your mind is at peace, your mental state and physical state will be in tune with the mind. Eczema manifests through the heart charka. Its psychological functions relate to love, balance and compassion. Emotional threats to this chakra include deep grief linked to past traumas, a fear of feeling emotions, a fear of rejection or abandonment resulting in a refusal to love again, lack of compassion and highly judgmental attitudes. Eczema is a result of the Root chakra and solar plexus chakra imbalances too therefore stress is the biggest cause of imbalance.

So healing the energy blockages and balancing the chakras I also suggest meditation, exercise and purifications. When the liver is weak, one knows that their solar plexus chakra is also out of balance leading to increase symptoms. Lastly, the throat chakra governs the endocrine system, the thyroid and parathyroid. The physical effects of a blockage in the throat chakra can result in eczema because frustration and mental distress from non-communication can increase signs and symptoms.

Daily Affirmation Given To Say Each Day:

New level of awareness: "I love myself and others. My skin is perfectly clear. I have no eczema at all"

Breathing

To boost Rachel's energy levels and have the ability to move forward. Extended exhale breathing is also beneficial as it allows the body to work towards an alkaline state as opposed to an acidic state. Alkalinity brings rejuvenation and relief to the body. For deep diaphragm breathing I suggested to be in a comfortable seated position, the breath is inhaled slowly and evenly from the diaphragm, through the nose.

Breathing is the simplest form of meditation and requires you to focus on your breathing. This type of meditation not only enlightens spiritually as you can connect to your inner self, but also makes the mind calmer, thus reducing anxiety, stress, depression, irritation, and anger.

Epsom Salts

This is excellent for relaxation and for drawing out pain and toxins of all kinds from the body.

Visualisation and Meditation

Rachel has spent a lot of energy worrying about things in life. Worry is counterproductive, and will not solve anything, but it will give a person a great deal of pain, and a gigantic headache. The opposite of worry, or fear, is faith. It can be helpful to visualize only what you want to experience, and to focus your thoughts as much as possible on the outcome that you would like to manifest, because your thoughts direct your reality. Use the power of visualization and meditation to relax and trust your own power to create the life you choose. Be grateful for the tests and challenges you have endured, because they have made you stronger, more creative and more resourceful. Instead of focusing on problems, ask for solutions to present themselves.

Every time you ask a question, the Universe provides an answer, so allow yourself to ask the right questions and focus on the right thoughts in order to get the answers, the ideas, the inspiration, the motivation and the outcomes that you desire to experience. Worry does not solve anything, and it only costs you vital energy and life force, and completely wastes your time. Worry will cause you to feel powerless and afraid, but every problem has a solution, if you are willing to shift your perspective in order to see it.

Positive Thinking

Negative emotions such as anger, resentment, bitterness, etc cause extreme tension in the body and release toxic chemicals. These negative emotions, if allowed to fester, will create terrible energy blocks in the body that can eventually manifest as disease of all kinds, especially cancer. Negative self-talk can cause chronic headaches. Self-criticism is a form of self-punishment. If you do not believe that you are a good person, then you will not believe that you deserve to feel good, or have good things or good experiences in life. It is best to be patient and loving with yourself under all circumstances, and to understand that sometimes we are hearing other people's judgments in our own head. People only judge others because of their own projections of pain and self-criticism. I talked with Rachel about allowing herself to relax and accept herself as she is, to love herself and allow herself to feel good and enjoy life. As you do this, your life will change to reflect your self-love and self-worth, allowing you to release your pain, self-punishment, and self-sabotage.

Pressure to Perform

Rachel felt a lot of pressure in her work and home life. This type of pressure caused Rachel to feel a great deal of tension or anxiety, and stopped her from breathing properly, which cuts off oxygen to the brain and can create headaches. This can also prevent her from being able to think or remember clearly. It is best to breathe, and relax, and envisage the outcome that you would want to experience. We looked at ways of visualising her winning, smiling, happy and at ease. Seeing everything flowing and going her way, with the desired results and outcome.

Calm the Mind

Rachel had so many thoughts and over-thinking can be very taxing and tiring for the brain. To help calm the mind I suggested it would be helpful to keep a journal, and to write down lists, especially when there are decisions to be made that are occupying their thoughts. Writing things down can get it out of one's mind, and once it is on paper, it can be easier to manage and to see clearly.

Perfectionist

Rachel was a perfectionist. The feeling of being driven or forcing oneself to do things one doesn't really want to do can create a lot of pressure and tension. Also, perfectionists are often very self-critical, and have a hard time forgiving themselves and others, which holds tension and negative emotions that increase toxicity in the body. No one and nothing on Earth is perfect - in fact, everything here is perfectly imperfect. There is no way to experience perfection other than accepting that everything is perfect as it is, including you. You can only do your best and give your best, and that must be good enough, or else your lack of self-acceptance and self-love will cause pain in many areas of life.

Diet and Exercise

Stretch; breathe fresh air; drink lots of pure water; move your body; walk; sweat to release toxins; breathe deeply to release through breath; eat whole organic foods as much as possible; take high quality vitamins and nutrients, especially essential fatty acids (fish oil, flax oil, etc).

Physical Relief

I suggested to rub the "web" of your hand between your thumb and forefinger; massage your temples in circles; rub your third eye in the middle of your forehead in gentle circles; massage the back of your neck and base of your cranium; massage the hinge of your jaw both on the outside and inside your mouth; cup your eyes with the palms of your hands; massage your sinuses above and below your eye sockets; rub your ears; use cold packs or hot compresses as needed, and a heating pad on your lower back this is great for intense physical relief you are mentally feeling every day.

Neem Leaves

Use of Neem leaves can be used as both oral and as topical treatment. It is recommended to chew 10-12 Neem leaves with water in the morning, but in modern society fresh Neem leaves might be hard to come by. So, capsule forms are also available. Taking the leaves or capsules for 10-15 days will reduce inflammation and infection in the stomach.

Nutrition

A diet rich in omega-3 fatty acids was recommended. This can be achieved by either fish oil supplements or by eating more cold water fish (e.g., mackerel, herring and salmon). This increases the acid level and really good to reduce the incidence of eczema.

Chamomile
A mild sedative, anti-inflammatory, and antibacterial, it improves digestion by relaxing the muscles throughout the gastrointestinal system and it can induce an overall sense of calm and well-being.

Dandelion
A leading remedy for detoxing the liver. It stimulates the flow of bile, a fluid that aids fat digestion, which is why it's used for liver and gallbladder disorders. Dandelion for its liver benefits dandelion is helpful for skin disorders.

Burdock Root
Helps to purify blood and restore the liver to aid in a restful sleep. The root reduces build-up of toxins in the skin resulting in boils and other skin disorders. It further helps gallbladder functions and stimulates the immune system.

Flaxseed Oil
Taken orally or applied externally often eases symptoms of eczema.

Meditation
There is nothing more powerful than meditation to reduce stress. Stress is one of the critical factors that aggravate eczema. Meditation should be practiced daily in a calming environment for at least 15-20 minutes at a time. Meditation benefits the body by lowering blood pressure, decrease heart and respiratory rate, increase blood flow, and increase the relaxation response.

Get Some Sunlight On Your Skin

Sunlight powers up our third, or solar plexus chakra. Getting 10-20 minutes of sunlight a day, especially on your stomach can improve your mood and digestion. Eczema is linked to 'not feeling powerful' so this is a nice self-love exercise. Don't do anything push the pause button. When you've suffered a serious loss, take a break. Take care of yourself and trust that the urge to get back at it will resurface.

Open Your Eyes

Fill your senses with music and the sights and sounds of nature. Visit museums and art galleries to get focused on the type of art you'll make when you're ready. Whatever touches your heart will help you heal. Being moved by what we see, hear, and feel leads to inspiration, and that gets us back to creating again, even when the darkness is so profound that we can't imagine it's possible.

Forget The Rules

Lose the rules about how to be a real artist. Don't worry about comparing yourself to your mother. Making art of any kind makes you real. Your creative process and your own style are what matters.

Find An Artistic Space That's Safe For You.

To get back to work we need physical space that also feels right emotionally. Give yourself permission to start small. If working at home doesn't work anymore, join an art club where you can make art every day or share a studio.

Lose The Guilt

Don't waste time feeling guilty for not making art – make some. Be your own B.A.F.F. (Best Artist Friend Forever). Praise yourself for each small achievement. When you're using a list, cross each completed task off and feel some pride as you do. Being kind to yourself helps you let go, relax, and get creative.

Recognise That You've Changed

Whether it's a month, a year, or 5 years since you produced your last piece of art, you're not the same person. You don't have to make the kind of art you used to make. Moving in a new direction may be the inspiration to get going again.

Remember The Bigger Vision

When you are ready, remember the world needs art and the world needs you. Gently, at your own pace, and always paying attention to what's most important to you, realise that people want to see your work. Your loss isn't any less, but art can be the path out of the darkness.

Rachel's Testimonial

Results didn't become better over-night, in fact, change was gradual and very subtle. A few years have passed since I had weekly "TOUCH" therapy, two, precisely. It has been a long journey. The eczema totally disappeared after nine months, and hasn't returned to date. The emotional signs of the imbalance have taken a little bit longer to heal.

I remember that the moment I understood this, I cried. I cried until my eyes hurt. Then I decided to take action, and it wasn't easy to uncover some hard truths, but it paid off in the long term.

I am off steroids and I am proud of the fact that I had the courage to stand by my beliefs and take a small risk. I tried the holistic route and it worked very well for me.

Because I had always had excellent skin, especially on the face, this created a great deal of additional stress and now I realise that the additional stress only encouraged greater areas of my face and neck to be affected. As well, my facial skin became excessively dry no matter what moisturiser I used, as did my hands, despite me being a heavy water drinker and consumer of organic only foods and drinks.

The year 2014, a good detox from the inside out was in order for certain. My skin needed to be hydrated constantly, this resulted in better sleep and being able to avoid the trap of obsessing over the problem. Eczema was reduced to a problem to be solved, and seemed somehow under control during my sessions with Sarah.

Baffling and frustrating are understatements that only touch the surface of how I felt as I tried to understand this entire situation, adding to the stress. I was not about to except taking steroids, being completely aware of the adverse health effects it has over time.

I took the liver detox remedy and I felt considerably better, and I began rebuilding my life little by little introducing the simple but effect lifestyle changes Sarah recommended. I realised I put so much pressure on myself personally when I was grieving I didn't realise I had nothing in my life except art, which was the one thing I was fighting with in my mind for all these years.

Today I can see that the severe stress I was under in 2014 set my skin up for trouble. Not only because of the cortisol released into the body during stress reactions, but because it depleted my immune system and also a big factor I never dealt with my inner emotions.

I don't believe there was only one culprit at work here, it was just a set of circumstances that made the situation come to a head. To reduce my stress levels, I've changed my lifestyle so I have time to meditate, sleep, spend time with friends, and stay fit. I also write a journal each day to unload my worries, fears and doubt. These days, if I feel an itch, I pause and ask 'what's below the surface – what is not being said?' Sarah has taught me well and I feel like I am now in touch with my inner emotions and instead of life ruling me I rule life.

After 6 months of seeing Sarah I picked up a paint brush and started to paint. I used to paint many people but I am now drawn to landscapes and natural art. I have a small studio I rent and commission my paintings. Every day I can take my pain and turn it into art painting my dreams!

Touch Therapy Conclusion

"Perhaps the blessing of eczema is to teach us to surrender to our natural sensitivity and to honour our intuition. To break the cycle of self-doubt and to STOP letting other people shape our lives"

Sarah Jones

About The Author

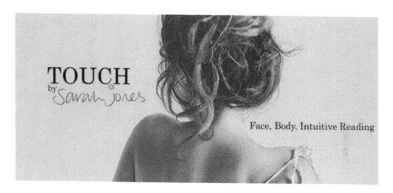

Sarah Jones – The UK's Leading Holistic & Intuitive Skin Expert

"Changing your skin…changing your life"

Sarah Jones is the UK's leading holistic expert. Using her unique gift of skin reading she is renowned for her signature TOUCH treatment. Sarah is a trained beauty therapist and has spent over 15 years in the holistic, wellness and beauty industry.

Sarah lives by the mantra that beauty on the outside begins with beauty on the inside; it is essential to our beauty that we lead a healthy lifestyle, an inner peace, positivity, confidence and overall balance. Sarah's vision is to restore health and wellbeing by awakening the beneficial 'healing energy' that resides within to nourish the body, emotions and soul.

Going beyond the traditional concept of beauty therapy, Sarah's philosophy stems from the connection between your complexion, feelings, self-confidence and power in your skin. Her biggest belief is skincare should compliment   the skincare products that we use - skin is only healed by soul searching within and healing the root cause.

Sarah states that in order to truly care for your skin you have to listen to it - a principle that is built on love, touch, gratitude and grounding; *"Admittedly the concept of listening to your skin may sound a little strange"*, she explains, *"but think about it along the same lines as trusting your intuition. Each person I treat with my signature TOUCH treatments has different needs and keys to wellness. There is never a one-size fits all rule."*

Sarah's TOUCH treatments take you on a profound and fascinating journey. Speaking of the treatments she offers Sarah comments:

"My treatments are designed to give you the information you need to get your skin – and your spirit – in shape. I tune into my client's skin and their life stories because beauty is more than just skin deep. While some people read crystal balls, I read your skin."

For more information please contact:

Lauren Lunn Farrow at Lunn Farrow Media

Email: Lauren@LunnFarrowMedia.com
Mobile: 07810 443 781

It Makes Sense When We Know Who We Really Are

I'm going to start at the age when I was forced to actually make decisions regarding my career. It's not that nothing juicy went on before then – and certainly there is plenty that is relevant to my journey – it's just that I'm not willing to share this with you until you at least buy me dinner... ;) I also don't want you to imagine that my 'career' is now wrapped up in a neat bow, pumping away and making total and complete sense. It really isn't and doesn't. I guess for me the journey has been about taking more ownership of my purpose and my authenticity in relation to this. I'm still very much in the process of creation but I've found a way to enjoy that and do it on my own terms.

So there I was, a soon-to-be Oxford graduate (Philosophy and French), delightfully weird and yet tragically unaware of this. I had not yet embraced the fact that I hate rules and get impatient with detail and therefore seeing as I could sometimes be a bit mouthy (and I loved the beauty of constructing a good argument), I thought it would be a great idea to become a barrister. It wasn't. I mean, I was ok at it really. I loved the human interest and the engagement with justice. But really and truly I did not embrace the Civil Procedure Rules one bit.

While all my friends were having fun barristering, I was asking my supervisor (previously known as 'master') annoying questions about the 'impact this would have on society'. This didn't endear me to him and he had this brilliant way of being perfectly polite but subtly contemptuous towards me the entire time. We all know someone with that skill. The barrister's chambers that I did my training in was staunchly refusing to modernise in any way - it has since disbanded - and they weren't really ready for someone with my personality and approach (friendly, talkative, open, not really interested in, well, the actual law). I used to dread Mondays so much that Sundays would see me plunge into doom. I'm glad to say that nowadays Sundays plunge me into embarrassingly low-brow consumption of TV and I thoroughly enjoy myself.

This mismatch between myself and my chosen career was evident from the start but I hadn't yet learned to listen to myself. From the very first day I had a sinking feeling. I couldn't bring myself to be enthusiastic about it to my friends and I remember being accused of negativity as I was supposed to be celebrating a great triumph and exciting new chapter.

If this had been my wedding I would have bolted for the door but instead I was solemnly going through the motions so as not to disappoint my guests. To be honest, the fact that I ever imagined I might thrive in a formal and hierarchical career structure is the first sign that I really did not know myself at all.

I have friends who manage to walk the line between what is expected of them and their true nature but I hadn't really learned that yet (it is questionable whether I have learned that at all). I was very, very confused at the obvious disdain for my contribution. My review stated (paraphrasing) "she's clever, great with clients, great with solicitors, motivated... she needs to develop a more professional edge in practice". I didn't realise that this was actually saying "she really isn't one of us".

Going back to the wedding analogy, it's a bit like someone saying you're really funny and clever but terrible at cooking and you think ah well of course they love having me as a wife! When actually they mean you are fundamentally terrible at your designated role. It's a complete distortion of your value and that can be hard to swallow. Not that I was a terrible lawyer, I could argue like the rest of them, it's just I was terrible at all the other bits and I really didn't see how my demeanour was relevant (I also never understood why my cooking capacity was relevant but that's another story).

I don't know if you have ever been in that situation yourself – where there are a lot of unwritten rules about behaviour and you keep accidentally flouting those rules. That would be fine if the hostility were direct and you could address the rules and negotiate them. But it's a lot harder to understand when the hostility is under the surface and you're left to figure out what is going on or try to negotiate the rules indirectly.

I used to be terrible at this. It can make you feel like you are somehow 'wrong' but you don't really know why. For me, I never followed a rule unless I understood its purpose and it somehow made sense to me but I wasn't aware of this yet – I would break rules unconsciously. I was just knocking around and naturally messing with the social scripts we all adopt (it makes things easier when we all know the rules of the game), maybe even throwing the script out completely, almost always making light of it, and definitely disrupting it in some way.

The reason I'm telling you this is because for me the hardest part of my whole journey was learning about who I am, the things I wanted to let go of and what to embrace. I now believe that authenticity is a person's greatest strength. It's not the rule breaking that actually gets you in trouble, it's trying to straddle the space between authenticity and what is expected of you.

I think if I walked into that job today just being myself without being afraid then we would either have negotiated a way of working with each other or we would have parted ways sooner. I would have been left less confused. It's hard to imagine that being honest gets you further (it can be really counterintuitive) but I swear I have always gone wrong the further I have strayed from my true thoughts, feelings and beliefs. I can't say I'm perfect at this – I still don't always speak my truth but it's liberating to be trying.

Another thing is, I sort of lied earlier when I said I wasn't terrible at being a lawyer. I became terrible at it because it was so out of alignment for me. There is nothing worse than directing your energies towards something that doesn't feel right - your performance drops and you also have to spend more energy trying to keep up with it. It just doesn't make any sense to live that way.

On the other hand, dropping out at the first sign of struggle, or because you are having a particularly boring, busy, or frustrating week can't be an option. We need to listen to our instincts on this. It's a subtle distinction and, from the outside, it might not be clear whether this is a momentary frustration or a misalignment with the soul. Get it wrong and it can either lead to us ignoring ourselves completely and carrying on regardless when really we need to get out or to jumping around from option to option at the first sign of discomfort.

I'm uncomfortable all the time now! All the time! Especially in the face of mundane tasks. Yawn. However, the underlying dread has gone. Only you will be able to tell the difference, it really is about trusting yourself.

So anyway, there I was, the world's least barristerish barrister who didn't even like rules anyway. But this wasn't the only reason I was struggling and really it's the other part that I want to talk about. My mum had died in an accident less than a year before I started law school and less than three years before I started my on the job legal training.

Not only was I traumatised, I was also living at home with my father who was traumatised from having watched the accident occur (my sister was at medical school – she has since left her profession too). I don't really know how to begin with the impact of a loss like this. Firstly, the loss of a parent at such a young age - 23 - and secondly under such violent and shocking circumstances. 23 is supposed to be an age of parties and festivals and romantic disasters (I had plenty of those).

It's a total mismatch from what I was going through. I think it was the emotional exhaustion that meant I wasn't able to ignore the signals about how I was living and what I was doing in my career. It obviously wasn't just my career either. Friendships and relationships were called into question – and believe me I made some epic mistakes there too. When they say "the rug was pulled out from under me" I now totally understand what that means. It's like you are flailing around trying to find something to grab onto and you can't see or hear clearly.

Once you are flat on your behind, you're in pain and bewildered and you're wondering how to get back up again. Mostly, you just want to lie back for a second. Except it's also like all your beliefs and understanding of the world tumble out of your ears on the way down and now you're left questioning everything.

So while everyone around me was enjoying being young, fresh and vibrant, I was plunged into a full on existential crisis while having to recover from a deep emotional wound. Oh, you can imagine what a great dinner party guest I was. A bundle of laughs. Actually, I was quite a good laugh at times because I would overcompensate by spending loads of money and trying to bribe people to stay out with me so I didn't have to go home and contemplate the innate fragility of our lives and how on earth I was going to survive without my mum (they really are like the air we breath, so necessary and yet half the time we barely notice this).

I don't even know what to tell you about how to survive bereavement. It's lonely. It's hard to explain to people how it's always under the surface but is also somehow difficult to grasp.

You just put one foot in front of the other for a very long time until you learn how to carry it better. You put down anything that is pointlessly exhausting. You probably try inadvisable ways of easing the pain and then abandon this when it makes things worse. You keep feeling it long after everyone expects it to have eased up. You never actually stop feeling it. And yet eventually life starts to creep back in, humour and light and trivialities, and you start to get interested in how to live properly again.

I can't tell you anything other than that I learned that I could endure more emotionally than I realised. And I decided to keep on going even when I really didn't want to, knowing that my future self would be grateful. And also because you actually pretty much have no choice anyway.

As you can imagine, I just did not have the willpower to keep going with something that didn't feel right for me so I left the law. It was a mutual decision between me and my - whatever the opposite of my biggest fan would be – my smallest fan? Biggest non-fan? My boss, in other words.

I went abroad and worked on child and women's rights issues. I didn't do this deliberately, it's just that people would ask me about them because I had been a lawyer. This is another really important point to make. You never actually leave things behind - they still form part of who you are and what you have to offer. People still take an interest in the fact I was a lawyer, I still use the skills I learned (I did actually learn things you know) and I still have doors opened for me because of my background – either because it is directly relevant or because it means I have something unique to offer.

A lot of people ask me about 'wasting' my time and investment on becoming a barrister but I don't see it like that. Firstly, life is way better when you allow yourself to make mistakes and 'waste' time. It's called experimentation and it's awesome. You can't really find your way until you at least start trying. Secondly, just because you don't do the same thing for life doesn't mean that experience has no value for you. Of course it does!

I mean - to bring it back to the marriage analogy once again for good measure – there is a difference between making the same mistake over and over again (although it does make for great celebrity gossip...). Making a mistake that is completely destructive, and having relationships that don't work out but that really teach you about how to love and be loved. The latter are hard but they are also opportunities.

Speaking of which, after all the volunteering abroad, I moved to Scotland and met a man. A cautionary tale of boy meets girl, girl thinks boy is answer to her prayers, boy is actually pathological liar. This was a break-up that hit me hard but it was also the gateway to my spiritual recovery.

I guess after the career change and the bereavement, although I had gone off on adventures and changed my external circumstances. I hadn't really even considered the internal work that I might need to do. It was only when I was knocked back again that I realised how unconscious I'd been – I think I was pretty much sleepwalking through life, probably as a result of being in survival mode for way longer than I expected.

It started small, with realising I needed to de-stress. I started to meditate and do yoga. I realised that I felt so much better for doing so. It opened up the space for me to become more conscious of my inner world. If you've ever done yoga you will be familiar with the emotions that can surface. Somebody advised me to try EFT. They had been experimenting with different forms of healing techniques and they said that it had been the most useful tool. It helps to let go of the unnecessary stuff that we carry and feel more balanced and free. I tried it myself and I was hooked.

Eventually, being a huge geek I jumped at the chance of doing a PhD with an academic I had come across during my Masters who I really admire (I still admire him but let's keep that between us, don't want to flatter him too much). I have just completed this PhD, which was on the emotional process of change as women leave prostitution and how we can support this in an emotionally intelligent way.

My journey was taking me on a path of really discovering how to support people, how people think and feel, and what it takes to transform your life (and having been through so many transitions myself I had really got my hands dirty with the process myself). In my private life, I was having fun with different spiritual and wellbeing activities but EFT was the backbone of my life, keeping me grounded and helping me to clear things that had been holding me back.

I decided to delve deeper into it and become a practitioner myself. I also started reading the book on Goddesses that inspired me so much I decided people needed to hear more about it. I began to develop the idea of Goddess Acumen, which is about embracing different aspects of our lives in all their fullness and potential and actually finding a way to be authentic.

I realised that many aspects of life that other people fear – sex, change, loss, purpose – were things that I now better understood. I felt I could help people to heal but also to lighten their load, explore and have fun with it (where this was possible). I also still do a lot of research and support other organisations to help people to make change. I work freelance, which is terrifying but also brilliant for my independent streak.

Sometimes I work too hard on things that aren't really what I would love to be doing. Sometimes I feel frustrated. Sometimes I worry about the future. But I do think that I've figured out my true purpose – combining adventure with the ability to help people transform – even though I am only just beginning to make that happen.

However, I am a lot better at listening to and trusting myself, have embraced my inner weirdness, and have learned how to navigate pain, loss, fear and even failure. I got fired from a job a couple of years ago (it was a part-time advocacy role) and I loved the fact that I had been a little bit humbled and also forced into doing something better.

I was no longer afraid of what that meant about me or even of the uncertainty it opened up because now the most important thing for me is to stay in alignment. Whenever I'm not, the universe has a funny way of letting me know about it – but I do always seem to survive.

Dr Helen Johnson

About The Author

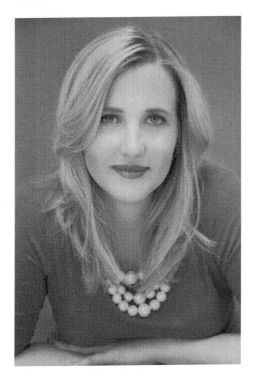

Dr Helen Johnson holds an undergraduate philosophy degree from the University of Oxford and a PhD in transforming lives. As the founder of Goddess Acumen, Helen uses therapeutic and personal development techniques to provide a cohesive approach to working with clients, enabling them to express their energies, find balance, manage change and transform their lives. Helen regularly gives talks and writes on the topics of emotional wellbeing, NLP, EFT and transformation. For further information on Goddess Acumen's one to one sessions, workshops and retreats in London and Barbados please visit:

Website: www.goddessacumen.com

Email helen@goddessacumen.com

Find Helen on Facebook and Twitter @goddessacumen

How I Overcame Depression & Suicidal Thoughts To Coaching Others Through Change & Trauma

As I sat in the shower cleaning the blood from the tiles, tears streamed down my face. Suicidal thoughts invaded my mind, and the emotions overwhelmed me. No matter how much I scrubbed the tiles, there was still blood. Except there wasn't – I was reliving having scrubbed the same shower after my brother's last suicide attempt.

Growing up, I remember an amazing life with my family that was full of love, fun and laughter. My parents were amazing role models in both life, love and business. I saw them work really hard in their businesses in London, while also making sure that we knew we were loved. I have fond memories of holidays around Europe having fun in the sun and exploring new places and people.

Although I didn't go through any trauma as a child, by the time I got to my teenage years I felt quite tortured in my mind. I had so many deep and meaningful questions about the meaning of life, but nobody around me seemed to think in the same way, so I had nobody to bounce these questions and ideas around with. I remember sitting in my bedroom trying to imagine dying and then not existing anymore – the thought of that really didn't make sense to me, but the thought of surviving in an infinite capacity was also overwhelming to me. These kinds of questions tortured my teenage brain and along with the dreaded teenage hormones, I felt like an outsider.

This longing for answers led me to taking it out on my body by restricting my intake of food and superficial cuts to my wrists. At age 17 I started studying psychology and philosophy at school in a bid to find some kind of answers and meaning. Psychology was definitely a piece of the puzzle for me, but philosophy tortured my brain even more – I felt like you could just talk meaninglessly about a theory you had and get a great mark if you talked long enough. But it never really answered any questions for me. I felt like I didn't know myself at all and I continued to feel this way for my entire teenage years. I went on to study a degree in psychology and a masters in forensic psychology, and I felt like I had found my "thing" - something I was good at and loved to read about.

At the age of 21 I met a group of friends who I consider to be my 'soul family.' From the minute that we met, we were having deep and meaningful conversations about the meaning of life, past lives, energy work, body wisdom and our past experiences. I finally felt as though I had found a tribe of people who I really connected with, who totally understood me and knew where I was coming from with my questions instead of thinking I was a freak.

One of them gave me a book to read called 'The Celestine Prophecy' and I was completely enthralled in it. Although it's put out there as a work of fiction, so much of it is based in fact, and it was an introduction to the world of energy. I felt as though this was another piece of the puzzle - I finally stopped questioning things so much and instead began opening up to receiving the answers.

Shortly after this I began studying Reiki, after a friend of mine gave me a Reiki treatment and began teaching me about the messages my body was trying to give me. I started teaching Reiki and a couple of years later I also started working as a life coach. I felt like I had really come home in terms of what I was doing in life and had a clear path ahead of me.

In 2007 I gained full-time work as a Probation Officer. I remember the day I started my training – 5th March 2007 – with such clarity, as it was the day a friend called me to tell me one of our best friends had committed suicide while on holiday in Australia. I was shocked – he had been the absolute life and soul of the party, and I just couldn't understand how this could be true.

A few months later I started a new relationship – one that would last three years and was built on a rocky foundation of manipulation and abuse. Halfway through this relationship my boyfriend at that time was diagnosed with bipolar disorder while locked in a psychiatric institution, after having four manic episodes with psychosis. When I reflect on these three years now it seems like it happened to another person, and it astounds me the bizarre things that would happen on a nearly daily basis.

During this relationship another friend of ours committed suicide, and shortly afterwards my brother had three extremely serious suicide attempts – the kind that he pulled off with such intelligence and planning that it's a miracle he's still here. The first was a "car accident," then he took an overdose, and the final time he cut his wrists and neck deeply then spent 48 hours bleeding in his London flat. Again, he had planned this meticulously so that he would die, but through a series of miraculous events my dad found him, nearly dead.

While my dad was at the hospital with my brother, I went to the flat with my boyfriend to start "operation clean up." I didn't want my dad to come back to the flat in the state it was in as it literally looked like a murder scene. I got into "work-mode" (which was really an avoidance tactic) and kept myself busy cleaning up the blood, making the place look as respectable as possible as my dad was spending the night there.

When I ran out of things to do, I sat on my brother's bed, facing the mirror. I suddenly felt the weight of his entire energy slam into my heart, and I wasn't able to avoid how I was feeling any longer.

My brother was diagnosed with depression and dysthymia (life-long sadness), and recovered well over the next few years with anti-depressants and psychotherapy, but mostly because he fell truly, madly and deeply in love with the amazing woman who would later become his wife and bear his children. Shortly after this event my boyfriend was hospitalised and diagnosed with bipolar, which was a relief to me as I believed he could get the help he needed and it wasn't all on my shoulders anymore. Or so I thought – the mental health system leaves a lot to be desired.

On his release back home, he was in major depression, and I became his carer. Everything felt so hard. I was still working as a Probation Officer, and on my arrival back home he would be there, waiting for me, opening my car door and dumping a barrage of all his negative thoughts onto me – the same thoughts he had day after day after day.

I tried so many different approaches to try and help him. After all, I was the "fixer" - I had all these tools in my toolbox and yet I felt none of them were working. I tried Reiki, coaching techniques, motivational interviewing, ignoring the problem, treading on eggshells, going to counselling with him, getting angry and frustrated with him, asking coaching questions, trying to put things into perspective, just being there for him and listening to him, but nothing seemed to make a difference. During this time we were still dealing with my brother and how we were recovering as a family.

After a year and a half of this, I slipped a disc in my back and was signed off work. At the time my biggest form of stress release and self-care had been exercise, but now I was forced into a situation where I couldn't do that. I was stuck at home with my boyfriend, being his carer but crying out inside for someone to care for me. I was burnt out and in constant physical and emotional pain.

For so long I had been the one who helped my friends get through their tough times, and now I was experiencing my own tough time, nobody knew what to do. It seemed to freak my friends out a bit that I was the one needing help. I tended to keep everything bottled up as over the years we had a lot of friends distance themselves from us due to my boyfriend's paranoid and psychotic behaviour.

After some time I just couldn't do it anymore. I realised that my back wasn't healing as well as it could due to the toxic energy I was spending my time in. After a frank conversation with my boyfriend, I realised he was in no way committed to his own recovery and that by me staying with him I was only enabling his behaviour. I packed my bags and moved to my parents for some much needed recuperation, and in doing so I realised that I had been staying with him due to a fear of him killing himself if I left due to his threats about this. It took only a couple of days for me to realise that I had fallen out of love with him a long time ago and I had allowed manipulation to keep me there.

Not long afterwards, I received a call from his sister saying he had jumped off the roof of our flat. It took me a long time to accept that this had been a suicide attempt, instead putting it down to paranoid thoughts – maybe he thought he was running from the police or someone who was out to kill him? I was in denial over that for a long time as I couldn't handle the guilt.

When living in my parent's house I was diagnosed with depression – again I tried to flat out deny this diagnosis, until my friends helped me to see there was no shame in me accepting that I had reactive depression after the years of trying to hold it all together for everyone else. I had been signed off work for a few months by this time and was still in constant pain. When I realised I couldn't even read a sentence of a book because my brain felt like it was melting, that's when I finally accepted I was in depression.

On a night out for dinner with my parents, I was engaged in superficial chit chat with my mum about the weather and the upcoming weekend. She asked me what I was doing that weekend (not much), and I asked her in return. She must have seen my vacant expression because she asked me to repeat back what she had said. To say I felt awful that I couldn't was an understatement. She then said to me "see? I told you, you don't listen."

I was absolutely gutted, ashamed and embarrassed. When you're knee deep in depression, you can barely remember your own name let alone a conversation. I was so ashamed I hadn't listened properly and I made it mean so many things about my nature like I was a terrible person, a bad daughter, worthless and not worth being around. I made a decision in that moment that my parents didn't want me around and so I left their home and moved into their flat in London – the same flat that my brother had attempted suicide in. In fact, I moved into his room, as he no longer lived there.

Here I was, living out of a bag at my parents as a 29-year-old woman with a failed relationship, broken body and a career on hold. A woman who was supposed to be able to help everyone else, who couldn't even fix herself. I got even deeper into depression after that, and that's when I found myself scrubbing the shower clean of blood – even though there was no blood there. I was recalling my brother's suicide attempt and the weight of the last few years was trampling on me. I was in a world of hurt at that point, and it was during my furious scrubbing of the shower that I began having thoughts pop into my head about how I would go about killing myself.

While I never really entertained those thoughts to the point where I made a proper plan, I knew in that moment how people can get to a place where they think the world is better off without them. Back then, I wished every morning that I woke up that I hadn't. But I never lost the spark of hope that I could get better. I was scared in that moment of what I might do to myself if I didn't take action in some way, and so I called my best friends – my soul family – who were at a house party on the other side of London. The absolute last thing I wanted to do was go to a party, but I knew I had to go and see them to talk. It felt like such a mission to drive an hour to the other side of London (when in depression an hour felt like a day, a day felt like a week), but I knew I had to do it.

I spent hours talking to my friends who helped me get a new perspective on things and helped me get my head out of it's dark space. Looking back on it now, it's no wonder I felt like this, living in the exact place where my brother attempted suicide. I was still carrying the weight of that around with me, and as an energy worker I was likely tapping into some of the thoughts he was having when he was at his lowest low.

My brother had watched me going downhill and was worried about me. I had told him about the conversation I'd had with my mum and he was upset with her for speaking to me like that. Only other people who have experienced depression know how damaging simple comments like that can be. He was concerned about the state I was in and wanted to help me get better, so he offered to pay for me to go on holiday somewhere so I could get away and get some sunshine. I reluctantly accepted his kind offer of help and it was the best thing I could have done for myself at the time.

I booked myself a week-long all inclusive trip to Turkey and soon found myself in the warm, healing sunshine. Although my usual nature is to be very outgoing and friendly, because I was in depression I was fearful of being away alone. Despite this, the desire to get away from it all and get better was stronger than my desire to keep myself isolated, and I knew the sunshine would be a powerful healer. I still couldn't read a book at that point – I love reading and with all the time off work I was frustrated that I couldn't get through any of my books. So I lay by the pool, in the sunshine, listening to Louise L Hay affirmations on repeat. After a couple of days of this, along with some good food and sleep, I realised I could read again and actually retain the information. I was so excited about this – it sounds so simple and yet for me it was my internal thermostat telling me I was starting to recover.

A group of girls who were on a girls holiday were sitting next to me at the pool and noticed I had been on my own, so they started chatting to me and took me under their wing. We had some great nights talking, laughing and drinking cocktails and I started to give myself permission to have fun again. The real me started to come back and I returned to London feeling more like my old self again. Shortly afterwards I went on holiday to Ibiza with my brother, his now-wife and a friend of his. I was about to move to Australia so this was a kind of "leaving treat" to myself. I'd planned for the last 10 years to move to Australia, and when I'd left my boyfriend one of the first things I did was buy my visa and one-way flight to Sydney.

During this holiday to Ibiza I felt so connected with my brother, and it began a powerful healing experience. I found myself in a club with him, watching him dance and have an amazing time, and I realised he had such a carefree energy about him – an energy that had never been with him his whole life before that. We had an amazing time together and he was so in love and happy, that I think I gave myself permission at that point to stop worrying about him, and finally start to heal the emotions I was holding on to about that time in our lives.

A few weeks later, after a whirlwind few leaving dinners, drinks and parties with my London soul family, I boarded a one-way flight to Sydney with nothing but two bags and a few boxes being shipped over, in search of a dream I had since I first travelled to Australia at age 19. I had the strangest experience when I had first travelled to Sydney ten years previously, where my heart felt like it slotted into place before I even got off the plane. I knew from that age that I would live in Australia and that it wasn't a case of if, but when. I was finally seeing that dream turn into a reality.

Within the first month of moving to Australia I met the love of my life while on a weekend trip to Perth, introduced to me by my best friends who were now living there. We got to know each other via a long-distance relationship and a few trips to Perth, but after two months we both decided it was time for me to book a one way flight there and start our lives together. I hadn't yet settled in Sydney and thought it was pointless trying to do so while my heart longed to be in Perth beside my man.

At the time of writing this, over six years have passed. In my first year in Australia I experienced depression and burnout again, and what I realised at that time was although I had felt as though I'd recovered, my brain hadn't quite corrected itself. This time I chucked everything at it – I was on a very low dose antidepressant for a few short months to get my head straight for counselling, where I started really digging deep into the last few years. I used various coaching techniques and did a lot of forgiveness work. I then trained as a Law of Attraction Coach and set up my business again in Perth as a Transformational Life Coach. I also started teaching Reiki workshops which became very successful. In 2015 I was granted permanent residency in Australia and a few weeks later I bought a block of land and started building my first home – my dream home by the ocean.

I left my full time job in April 2016 to pursue my business full time. We moved into our home a few weeks later and my partner proposed on our first night there. To say that I am now living the life of my dreams is a huge understatement – everything I used to dream about having in my life is now my reality and I pinch myself when I look out at the beautiful, magnificent ocean from our kitchen.

I had to do a hell of a lot of personal development to get myself here. I've done multiple courses, trained as a coach, and worked through my past and my shadow self-using a range of different tools including NLP (neuro-linguistic programming), EFT (emotional freedom technique), forgiveness work, and techniques rooted in the law of attraction, among others. There is always more to do, and I do work on myself every day. I'm totally committed to walking my talk.

There are so many people in this world who are feeling hollow, stuck and disconnected. Although I had started coaching in 2008, it was only in 2016 that I really opened up to my niche, those people that I am destined to help.

I now spend my days coaching and mentoring others who are currently where I used to be, feeling depressed and suicidal, or going through a major life change that they are struggling to cope with. I absolutely love what I do and am so grateful for all my past experiences as overcoming this adversity has allowed me to truly grow into the truth of who I am, and allowed me to find my path in life.

I am passionate about doing my bit to reduce to global suicide rate because suicide is completely preventable. I also welcome sharing my story with others because if I can overcome this, then others can too.

Carly Evans

About The Author

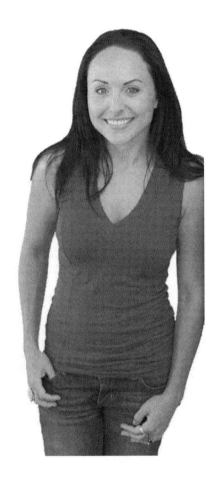

Carly Evans is the founder of Coach Carly and Phoenix Transformation. She is a Transformational Life Coach, Reiki

Teacher and energy practitioner who is based in Perth, Australia, but who works globally. She launched an online program called From Surviving To Thriving to support others overcome their own adversity.

To find out more about Carly visit:

www.coachcarly.com

www.facebook.com/coachcarlyevans

www.facebook.com/phoenixtransformation

Twitter: @coachcarlyevans

Instagram: achcarlyevans

Carly Evans aka Coach Carly

GET YOUR FREE E BOOK AT www.coachcarly.com

Transformational Life & Body Coach (certified through the Inspired Spirit Coaching Academy)

Contributing Author in the internationally bestselling Adventures in Manifesting series (Soulful Relationships)

Reiki Master Teacher

Surviving & Thriving After Narcissistic Abuse

This is a story of surviving narcissistic abuse and how I use my incredibly traumatic experience with it to help others.

Before I get to that, let me tell you a little bit about who I am. I am a happy, kind-hearted, caring, confident and bubbly introvert. In recent years I have dedicated my life to serving others and helping them overcome emotionally tumultuous experiences that linger and haunt them for a long time after the event.

At this point you may be wondering why. For someone who appears outwardly like a happy, kind-hearted, confident and bubbly person, I have certainly had my challenges over the years – and it wasn't an easy process to evolve into who I am today.

When I was a little girl I grew up in a small town in country Australia with a *big* imagination. I was popular and good at everything I tried. And for as long as I can remember, I was a good girl who tried to do exactly as she was told when she was told to do it.

Everything changed just after I turned 11.

That was when my parents moved me from all my friends and the surroundings I knew to the city. And I quickly turned into the country kid outcast. I was diagnosed with Scoliosis when I was 13,

I had a big, ugly, fibreglass back brace from 14 to 15, and then had the surgery at 16.

I was bullied and tormented relentlessly, from girls at the posh private girls' school I attended and boys from a nearby school – some of who are trying to find out how I'm doing now and are still apologising to me … and I'm in my 30s! I definitely think it shaped my life – but not necessarily in a bad way – and while they remember who I am, I don't remember any of them. Not by face or name.

When I was 17 I was diagnosed with acute depression following many years of bullying. I had been in and out of hospitals and was in such a bad way emotionally that I was told I'd be on medication for the rest of my life. "It's like diabetes – your brain just naturally doesn't produce serotonin, like the pancreas doesn't produce insulin", I was told.

When I was 22, I started to change my life around. I managed to take myself off medication completely – and much to the amazement of my psychologist and people around me: I improved almost immediately. I believe the reason I improved so quickly was because I knew without the medication, I would be forced to take action. And I did! I started taking responsibility for my life and started taking the steps I needed to in order to make a real difference to my life.

I've never needed to return to medication.

Overcoming all of that was probably my greatest achievement. Until I turned 30.

When I was 30 years old I fell in love with a man who was anything but what I would've chosen for myself. Harry[1] was 15 years older than me, I didn't find him physically attractive at all, he had two children and he was separated from his wife. But he had this way of making me feel special like no one else ever had.

We met at work – he was one of my managers – and no matter what I produced, he always made it seem like it was a masterpiece. He'd go around making a big deal about it to anyone who would listen – "Sarah did this – doesn't it look great? She's so much better than the last marketing girl". It made me feel good.

I would meet him early (before I started work) just to spend time with him. One day he stopped me as I was walking out of his office to tell me, very emotionally, that he and his wife had separated and that I was the only person he felt he could tell. We were just friends, but of course I'd support him.

After that he wanted to spend more time with me. He would turn up at my apartment unannounced with a takeaway bag and dinner. He didn't ask what I wanted – just ordered. It was always amazing too! The first time he did it he brought me alcohol. It was my favourite and he had only seen me drink it once. He was

---

[1] Some names and identifying details have been changed to protect the privacy of individuals.

really attentive and just really cared about every little detail about me. He also started reading every blog post I'd ever written and started focusing our conversation on it.

My boyfriend at the time never would've done that for me – but ironically he was someone I thought I always wanted. He was my age, exceptionally good looking and he always pushed me to be independent. He was extremely introverted so if we did spend time together it was very limited and I generally had to fit in with that.

But for the first time, I felt as though I could relax with Harry. Being myself was always more than good enough – even on an off day!

Within two weeks I had abruptly left my boyfriend. "Something is broken and we can't fix it" I told him – exactly as Harry had told me to say.

Everything was so easy with Harry. He made even the simplest things – spending time together – feel so important and so amazing. And other people noticed the special magic too. Although we were inseparable, people would stop us in the street and ask to take a photo of us together because they had "never witnessed a love like this before". It was like a Hollywood movie!

Hopefully they never do again...

Because what I didn't know at the time, was that Harry had Narcissistic Personality Disorder and perhaps the reason our romance felt like a Hollywood movie was because it was. It wasn't real – it was learned. And at the time I was being groomed and lulled into a very dangerous relationship.

A week after we started seeing each other I was getting forced out of the apartment I was living in. I was living with a girl who just didn't like him. So I moved out on my own, as Harry suggested – it wasn't that much more expensive. Within days of moving into my own place, Harry had moved in with me.

We lived together in a studio apartment for six months and never argued. I paid rent and bills, and he paid for food – because although he earned three times what I did, he was anticipating child support. It was literally perfect. Every day we would write love notes to each other on a whiteboard. During the day we exchanged thousands of text messages – even when we worked together, although I quickly left my job because I was scared living and working together would be too much. Even after that it felt like we loved each other more and more each day.

So I thought...

One day Harry said he needed his own space. And I encouraged it. He wanted to show his kids that he was independent and could be on his own. He started inspecting properties, even asking me to go – while his kids were there to help him choose. He ended up taking a studio one level above mine – so we could still see each other all the time. It was about six months in, and only a week or two after he moved in, a friend from my previous workplace (where I'd met him) had tried to warn me about him.

He said Harry was trying to work it out with his ex-wife. I didn't believe it. I immediately confronted Harry. I'll never forget his instant explosive anger. He was at work at the time and screaming about how the person who warned me just wanted to break us up so he could have me for himself. And then he suggested we were already involved. I was shattered and scared of losing Harry. I reassured him that it was ok and he said that was lucky because the person who told me is a thief and he lies "because that's what thieves do". That was our first fight.

The next week my friend was fired for stealing.

Looking back, I could almost swear it was a set up, but at the time it just appeared to be more evidence that Harry would never lie to me and I shouldn't doubt him.

About a month later I got a call from Harry – he sounded worried. "My wife wants to talk to you," he said.

"So let her – I have nothing to hide," I responded. I knew she knew about us, because he told me he had spoken to her about me.

The next day I was on the phone to her. She told me he'd never left her and they were still very much married and together. I couldn't get my head around it. The entire world I knew turned on its head. I remember literally feeling dizzy as my world turned on its head at the betrayal.

Even now that I'm well out of it, I don't know how that was possible. He was living with me, I didn't dream that – but I questioned it. I questioned my entire grip on reality. When it got too much, I demanded to talk with him (he was with her then) but she refused to put him on the phone. He wouldn't take my calls and he pretty much vanished. I couldn't contact him at all. His absence, and the overwhelming pain, were the only two ways that I could I acknowledge that my experience was real and it wasn't all in my head.

My day-to-day functioning disintegrated.

I went to work the next day, but couldn't work to my usual standard. I got in trouble by a senior manager and took a break to get my head back together. As I walked back to work I saw him driving towards our apartment. He pulled over and I got in. The connection was instant. We were both crying. I begged him to spend the afternoon with me and he agreed. I sent a text to my manager saying I wasn't feeling well and was going home. I also contacted a friend to bring me my bag. He brought it up and when he got there was really worried: "Sarah – get out of the car," he said, holding the bag behind his back.

"I'm fine – I'm ok!" I sobbed, as I got out of the car and ran and snatched the bag and got back in the car.

We drove off.

Once we returned home Harry told me he was going back to his wife.

Within half an hour, he was gone again.

I was physically sick. I had a complete breakdown.

At the time, I deluded myself into thinking it was just another "toxic relationship" … and I wrote an article on my blog about toxic relationships. Trying to help others in this situation. http://sarahjwebb.com/all-about-toxic-relationships-and-how-to-let-go/

I'm not easily misled. I've had boyfriends before. I've been cheated on before. But this was overwhelming because I completely questioned my entire reality. Did I dream it?

I couldn't function at all. I didn't contact work. I just planned to never go back. I was so humiliated. I couldn't make sense of anything. And I felt as though I couldn't talk to anyone because no one would get it. They'd just think it's just a break up – get over it, right?

Fortunately my manager saw through it, and knew it was symptoms of something more serious. She was very patient and negotiated with the human resources department on my behalf. When I was ready, I could return part time until I could take on more pressure. I agreed, and committed myself to doing whatever it would take to recover.

I moved back to my parent's house.

Within days Harry was contacting me again. And within the week I was moved back home and we were seeing each other again. It felt like he'd never left. He told me she was threatening to kill herself. And when he told her he wanted to be with me, she started slashing at her arms and wrists in front of him, his brother and their youngest child. She was taken to hospital and that night he was back next to me – like nothing had happened.

That was when he told me his wife wanted to get an AVO (Apprehended Domestic Violence Order) against me. "She can't! I haven't done anything wrong!" I protested. I couldn't understand it.

When she got out of hospital she tried calling him 300 times. He asked me to watch her using a GPS tracker to ensure we were both safe and clear of her. We went to the police and he just asked them to call her to tell her to stop calling.

The calls stopped.

It was like she was finally gone. But still something sinister hung in the air. Something wasn't quite right.

For the next little while he left his phone out. He was open about everything. And he did everything he could to get my trust back. It didn't take long for the attachment to take hold again ... It also didn't take long before I felt as though I was losing him again – as I noticed he started taking his phone with him every time he went to the bathroom. This time I wasn't having any of it. "No! I will leave you!"

I thought I was in control ... I couldn't have been further from it.

He started threatening me with an AVO again – this time saying if I left him he had a friend high up in the police force who would help him get it – and he would seek the highest order against me. I didn't believe he could or would – I'd never even had a parking ticket before. It scared me and I wanted to do the right thing and avoid it, so I stayed with him and this horrible, chaotic limbo became my life for a few more months.

It was constant fighting and I had to attend a friend's wedding in another state. He threatened to follow me and make it hell. Sure enough, the morning I left he came out in front of my family and I with his bag and walked up the road. The people at the desk wouldn't tell me if he was going to be on my flight despite my desperation and tears. It was horrible – I was constantly watching over my back.

Christmas was a nightmare – he vanished again.

I started seeing other people and he started stalking me. He would come up out of nowhere and tell me who he saw me with, describe what they were wearing and tell me where we went. He called me a whore and accused me of going with anyone. Then started demanding his stuff back, that he'd left at my apartment – even things he'd given me, like a phone charger – and telling me to leave it by his car. All of a sudden he was angry at me, like I had done something wrong. At the same time he would tell me to leave things at his car, he would tell me to stay away from his car – it was totally confusing.

And that's when I told him it was over. I didn't care anymore. The next day while I was on my lunch break, the police called. His wife had lodged a complaint against me.

I burst into tears and asked them to help me and they told me if I did anything else I would be arrested. At the same time, this made me think he didn't lie that she really had lost it — and I couldn't help but feel sorry for her for being so easily manipulated.

I stopped sleeping and started having nightmares.

When I'd see Harry around our apartment block he became physically abusive. He started grabbing and shoving me, slapped me in the face, spat on me … I took photos of the bruises on my arm in case I ever needed evidence. At the time, I made a complaint and the police offered to put an AVO in place against him when I finally went to them but I thought about his children and how manipulative he is — I'd seen him get out of trouble with the police before, and it was like he knew he'd get away with me — and I decided I couldn't proceed.

The senior policeman walked out of the room muttering "It's just a piece of paper anyway", and I was alone with a junior who said very quietly "If you don't get one against him, he will get one against you." I started crying — I didn't want to harm him, I didn't want anything in place, I just wanted things to be different.

One morning I caught Harry at his car as he was going to work and stood in front of it trying to force him to stop and talk to me so we could sort something out and at least be civil. He turned the car on and started driving forward into me. I wasn't scared at the time – perhaps too angry to be scared. Too addicted to him to care that he could kill me. But it did significantly impact me a few weeks on.

The next day I saw Harry in the carpark of our apartment and he acted like nothing had happened. He asked me to come up to his apartment later. As I got to the door he went crazy: "Why are you here? What are you doing? Leave or I'll call the police." And he started dialling. I thought maybe he had a mental illness I didn't know about. He did this a few times saying "Call me later" and I'd say "But you've blocked me", "It's ok – I just don't want my wife seeing it's you, call me on my private number". So I did … and I'd call and call and call – no answer. On the odd occasion he did answer, he'd say something muffled and hang up, so I'd try ringing again to see if he'd talk. He didn't.

One day I went on a bike ride with a friend. As we were leaving, we saw him in the garage. My friend just shook his head – but I knew this would mean trouble. He never liked seeing me with anyone else. That afternoon I was rushing to get somewhere when I noticed I had a letter on the windshield of my car. It was him saying how much I'd "hurt" him. I then tried to contact him again to apologise. Once again he'd answer and then nothing. I wanted to inconvenience him too, so I walked over to his car and lifted his windscreen wiper blades out of sheer frustration.

A couple of days later I decided to completely stop contact. I wouldn't respond at all. I was tired of being up and down – a New Year was coming and I was determined that he wouldn't be part of it.

So there I was on New Year's Eve, getting ready in front of my mirror when my intercom went. I had lived in my apartment for almost a year and that intercom had never buzzed. It was the police … the same police station where I had been to seek help only the week before. They were there to serve *me* with an AVO on his behalf. The grounds were "harassment" and the order was requested for a two-year period. The only factual thing on there was that I'd lifted his windscreen wiper blades – the rest was a lie. It was only then, seeing it in black and white, and seeing that he could lie to the police – that I realised he lied. All the time.

I thought about not going to court but that meant the order would be in place. I watched The Hunger Games on repeat to try to learn courage. I was backed into a corner – because my options were:

1. Confess with admissions, it goes in place
2. Confess without admissions, it goes in place
3. Fight it – which means turning up three more times to see him, missing work and paying $3,000 for the legal fees.

Trying to find a family lawyer over the Christmas period was nearly impossible. I somehow managed to find two – which allowed for a second opinion on the case. Standing by my New Years resolutions I decided there was only one option – not to play his game anymore.

By the time I returned to work after the Christmas holidays, I'd dropped two dress sizes. Some people asked how I did it, some people just expressed their concern for me. I was so ashamed, I only told my manager and my friend who took my bag to me that day.

My parents and best friend (a guy that Harry didn't like because he always felt threatened by him) stood by my side. My best friend held my hand the entire time. I wouldn't look at Harry, not even in his direction. My resolution was that I wouldn't see him that year. So he started pacing the halls until he literally backed all of us into a corner at a fire escape.

When my barrister appeared, I got to talk to him before we went into the courtroom. We had agreed that he would speak, all I needed to do was attend. I knew this would anger Harry because I personally was not consenting – and that's what he really wanted. Before we left the consultation room, I asked if he could request contact clauses to be put in. He smirked at me "I don't think that'll be necessary, do you?" I just stayed quiet. He went on to tell me how it would work against me – because if I was found to contact him, then I'd be facing two years jail time. I felt overwhelming panic at the thought.

I couldn't understand it – so what he was saying was that according to our laws an AVO doesn't stop you from calling or seeing the person, and if you want that "extra level of protection" something very serious has to have happened. And yet – if you go to a psychologist or psychiatrist about a toxic or abusive relationship, the first thing they advise is to cut contact.

In the hearing, all I had to do was stand up a couple of times. I didn't speak. The lady next to me gasped in horror as I stood, that I was the "perpetrator". I could tell the magistrate knew something wasn't right – but I knew if I wasn't going to defend myself there was nothing they could do about it either.

It was my choice

The AVO was put in place against me for six months (not the two years he asked for) and after the hearing a senior sergeant representing him approached me and my parents. He tried to appear reasonable and said "Sweetheart, next time come and see me, don't let it get to this..." I stepped back and all I could manage was: "I did! I was there ... I did..."

Didn't they look at their records? Didn't they see that this was *exactly* what he had threatened me with? Oh but that's right, it's not a threat of violence or anything that will harm me so not to be taken seriously.

After the hearing I moved house. That same day I moved into a really nice, high-security, luxury apartment where I knew I would be safe. He could go back to his wife – I didn't care – I just wanted my life back and to feel safe again. All I cared about was regaining my peace and freedom.

As I left the court, my friend and I danced in the street with sheer relief. It was over! It was *finally* over. I was FREE!

I had a new phone (because I worried my ex had bugged my old phone), I blocked him from all my social media and my emails and

I moved into my beautiful apartment and I prepared to start again. What I didn't expect were the suffer symptoms of Complex Post Traumatic Stress Disorder (C-PTSD). I started carrying out bizarre rituals, such as checking my locks in order, then checking them again to make sure everything was locked. I couldn't sleep until I closed my door and put a pillow against it. I suffered flashbacks and had nightmares. I could hardly cross a road because I was paranoid he would come out of nowhere and mow me down… or he would organise for someone else to do it for him.

Three days after the court hearing it was my birthday.

I was at my computer and opened my email to see what birthday messages I had received. Sure enough there was one from him. "Happy Birthday". I hadn't blocked him properly. That was when I realised there was something seriously wrong with him and that he did deliberately try to hurt me. I fell to the ground and sobbed and sobbed. I decided not to respond but knew it would only be a matter of time before he would retaliate.

I spent that afternoon writing an article for my blog (I'd been keeping it religiously for two years). It was about how to stop someone controlling you with all my hindsight. The article was instantly popular – apparently people had been looking for this information … including him – because shortly after it was published, he commented. He tried to expose me for receiving the AVO saying I "deserved" it – an ironic comment seeing as I'd had no contact with him, he'd wished me happy birthday and was now commenting on my blog.

What I didn't know as that I wasn't alone. Six weeks after I was served with this AVO a report was released about other women in New South Wales, Australia who had also been the victim of domestic violence and served with a manipulated protection order. One of the lawyers I saw said it was common and he saw "the mistress" served all the time:

"The study findings include that over two-thirds of our women clients defending AVOs reported that they were the victims of violence in their relationships. Fewer than 40% of these clients had a final AVO made against them when the case came before the court. Many of the women defending AVOs reported that when police had been called after a violent incident, they felt that their version of events had not been viewed as credible compared with the other party, due to the circumstances of their heightened stress and anxiety."[2]

A couple of days later my old manager (from the workplace where I met Harry) had commented on my blog Facebook page inferring that I was a liar. I hadn't seen him or had anything to do with him in the past year. I was amidst a narcissistic smear campaign.

The following week a mysterious man requested my friendship on Facebook. Philip Matthews. I'm fairly savvy when it comes to technology, and what my ex didn't realise I could search Facebook by email address. I entered the email address that he

---

[2] http://www.wlsnsw.org.au/wp-content/uploads/womendefAVOsreport.pdf

used to comment on my blog and sure enough, up popped Philip Matthews.

At the time I wasn't leaving my apartment at all – I decided I wasn't going to leave my apartment so long as the order was in place. My biggest concern was that if he saw me, he would manipulate what happened and have me put in jail. I would be in the same helpless position I felt like I was in now.

After an entire month, the AVO still hadn't arrived in the mail. Did I dream that too?

I knew it was only a matter of time before he came for me again, so I compiled my evidence and all the screenshots I needed. I had all the evidence I needed to prove that in fact *he* was stalking me and not the other way around.

Since I had moved house, I had been to the police station three times to see the senior constable I had met in court, after he had invited me to see me if there was an issue, before it escalated. He wouldn't do anything. In fact, I was told I was an attractive girl and I should just "move on". I was also told I was on "some kind of revenge mission".

Finally I went directly to the magistrate for support – and while I was there, I requested a copy of my AVO. The reason I had never received it was that my address was completely incorrect – after my barrister had clearly spelt it out. Was that incompetence? What if I really did need an order against me?

Although I realised perhaps this piece of paper really wouldn't protect me at all, I thought it was still worth having something at the court about it. It turns out, the magistrate have a message-only system. You leave a message with the report and they call you back when it suits them. You also only have a couple of tiny boxes to fill in with all the details of your story and your evidence.

It took two very long days for the magistrate to finally call me back.

I was at work so I snuck into a small office to take the call. It had been the longest two days of my life and I was so relieved when I heard it was them. Finally, something was going to happen – they would protect me – and I could feel safe again.

But instead I heard the magistrate say I didn't have any evidence they could go on. In fact, the evidence I had presented could be considered as *cyberstalking*. That meant I was in breach of my AVO for stalking and would be facing two years jail time. The magistrate acted like I was a complete waste of time.

I managed to get through the rest of the day in complete numbness.

I was on autopilot. I didn't speak to anyone. I thought it was a matter of time before the police would come for me to take me to jail. In fact, I thought they'd probably turn up at my work at any moment.

When I arrived home that afternoon, I sat on my couch for hours in silence.

I didn't turn on the TV.

I wasn't thinking.

I just sat there.

Numb.

Then I carefully carried out my plan to end my life.

The next day, I blinked my eyes open following my suicide attempt.

I felt really sick.

I started crying.

I felt so helpless.

"Sarah, what are you going to do?" I asked myself, out loud.

And I have no idea where it came from but a voice within said "I'm going to recover, I'm going to get better and I'm going to make sure this *never* happens to anyone else!"

So, I focused on all my energy into my recovery.

I tried to stay forward-focused. I took it moment to moment, and soon I could take it day by day, but nothing was easy.

I re-negotiated my hours at work so I could leave work during daylight hours and so he wouldn't be able to wait for me or follow me. I then had people at work complaining that it wasn't fair.

But still, I concentrated forward.

For months I struggled to communicate with people because I had short-term memory loss (associated with C-PTSD). I'd start saying something and then pause, and I'd have absolutely no recollection of what the conversation was about. Sometimes I humiliated myself even more by trying to guess what we were talking about – and I'd finish the sentence talking about something completely different to what we started talking about.

That took almost a year to completely recover from so I could have conversations again.

One of the ways I worked to get my memory back was I decided to study life coaching. I had been thinking about it for years but it was never the right time. As I started studying, I realised it could be used to help other people like me – with simple practical steps to help people get out and move forward.

I started campaigning that AVOs need to come with mandatory contact clauses for both parties – meaning if either party break the order they would be fined, holding them both accountable. I wanted psychologists to be involved with the process – and to implement mandatory counselling for six weeks to both parties following an order being put in place. But no matter what solutions I came up with, they fell on deaf ears. More frustrating was the fact that it's a global issue and every country has different laws.

I wanted these changes to be implemented globally.

That's when I decided, that if I couldn't help change the systems on a global scale, then I would work with them and find a way to support people around them. As our systems currently stand, men and women die every day as a result of domestic violence partnerships – and previously violent partners.

And so as soon as I graduated, I opened my company Relationship Free and took blogs and diary entries and all my notes from my own therapy that I'd received and I put together a program that will help other people heal from narcissistic abuse.

I had Relationship Free for a few years but it kept me stuck. Most clients wanted free support and I felt like it was attached to him. So early in 2016, I made the bold move to open a business in my full name.

I knew it would be a risk that he could find me again but Relationship Free was born out of fear – it kept me hidden, whereas Sarah J Webb was born from courage and it illuminates the importance of being self-confident and independent following emotional trauma – and that it is possible as you take *a journey to a better you*.

My greatest achievement is now transforming something so ugly, a blotch on my record and overwhelming fear, into a positive way to help others.

It was a natural progression for me to take something negative and transform it into a positive. That AVO is now not something I'm ashamed of, it's my Diploma of Narcissistic Abuse, because without it, I wouldn't do what I do today.

Sarah J Webb

About The Author

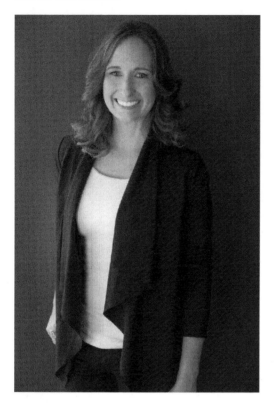

Sarah J Webb is a qualified life coach, NLP Practitioner, trauma counsellor and hypnotherapist.

Having overcome years of bullying, toxic relationships, domestic violence, a fear of abandonment, love addiction and depression, Sarah became passionate about supporting men and women on a journey to becoming a better version of themselves.

It was after her experience with domestic violence that Sarah left her career in marketing to assist targets of toxic and abusive relationships to break the attachment to an experience or person that is hurting them, and recovery.

Sarah works with people to offer simple practical steps they can take to move forward from where they are today and fast-track the healing process so that they can achieve their biggest goals tomorrow.

Forward thinking, forward focused and forward moving in all approaches, all of Sarah's products and services are designed to focus on what individuals can do now to succeed, feel great and get the best out of life.

If you'd like to find out more about Sarah's you can find her on the following:

My website is: http://www.sarahjwebb.com

Facebook: www.facebook.com/iamsarahjwebb

Twitter: https://twitter.com/SarahWebbCoach

LinkedIn: https://www.linkedin.com/in/sarah-webb-5b788145

Instagram: https://www.instagram.com/ajourneytoabetteryou/

Pinterest: https://au.pinterest.com/SarahJWebbCoach/

YouTube Channel: www.youtube.com/c/sarahjwebb

Facing Trauma Head On....

No one ever thinks that something bad will ever happen to them, why would we?

I was living a happy and content life with my wife of 358 days. We lived in a two-story place on the North Shore in Sydney, Australia. Between the both of us we had good jobs and lived a pretty comfortable lifestyle. To some extent we probably lived and had more stuff than we required. We were able to travel regularly where ever we wanted to go and buy the things that, well, we just wanted to have but didn't really need. That's life isn't it though?

The place we lived in had 4 bedrooms, 3 bathrooms, double lock up garage, a yard, the only thing that was missing at the time was a four-legged creature or a child to add to the family which we had been planning and talked about.

It was 1 week to our 1st year wedding anniversary, it was no different to any other Saturday that we had spent together over the last 5 years or so but this day Saturday 26th February 2012 will forever be etched in my head and my life. This is my story that not only affected me but many others on different levels, my personal struggles, and battles that I've faced during the last four and a half years but also the steps along the way that have helped me during this time to get me to where I am today. I couldn't have thought of a better title for this book when I was asked to contribute a chapter towards it. IF I CAN, YOU CAN.

No matter what your circumstances or position in life, if you can learn just one thing from my situation and story, hopefully you will be able to take that first step of action whether it be to help yourself or someone else who is going through difficult times.

What Happened

To give you a bit of a background on what I'm about to talk about in this chapter, you need to know that I was once very athletic and sporty in my younger years and competed at quite a high level. Because of all that wear and tear on my body due to the constant training and playing of sport my body was trying to tell me stop doing this or slow down. After 4 knee reconstructions, ankle reconstruction, hand surgery and numerous fractured bones in my ankles I kind of got the message. Due to all these operations and me wanting to get back into some form exercise again as well as trying to realign all my body parts, I decided to go and see an exercise physiologist which really is a more qualified version of a personal trainer who could assist me with this process in moving forward.

It was the day of my assessment with the personal trainer and for some reason I asked my wife at the time to come along with me as I wasn't particularly feeling that well and didn't really want to drive. Plus she was also thinking about getting back into exercise with a personal trainer also. As it was only an assessment, we were only doing basic things such as cardio to start with to see my level of endurance followed next by strength.

So, 15 minutes into my assessment I had done an initial set of bench presses as a warm up. What happens next is not a joke and may take some time to digest as people still can't fathom it. After having done my initial warm up bench press set the trainer adds more weight to the bar, in-between this I'm waiting for him lying on the bench when all of a sudden I feel this thud, followed by a

'What The Heck just happened?' I wake up a few seconds later to see my white shorts now red, blood pouring out everywhere and my jaw and mouth in considerable amount of pain while trying to work out what just happened. Meanwhile seeing my wife run over to me and yelling at the trainer: "what did you do?"

What happened was that after he had put the weights on the bar he went to lift it up accidentally with one hand and it slipped out and fell onto my face, more so in-between my mouth and chin. To look at it in a positive light if it had of been 1 inch higher it would have shattered my whole mouth, 2 inches higher and it crushes my nose which would have resulted in a whole face reconstruction, a few inches lower and it squashes my throat which, had that happened, I most likely wouldn't be writing about this in all honesty. So, landing just below my mouth and opening up a hole that went all the way through and crushing my jaw wasn't a bad result I guess looking back on it now.

Battles I Encountered

Having suffered and experienced quite a traumatic accident like that explained above then what was to come and the after effects of it all would test any persons resolve. This next little section I will briefly go into other battles I faced and went through over the last 4 years.

Firstly, I had the initial injuries suffered that I knew of within the first few weeks of the accident happening. Upon the bench press bar hitting my face it created a nice gash and hole below my mouth and above my chin in that little crease part which was gushing out blood. The first steps were to get the claret stopped and have that crater stitched up which at the time the doctor didn't realise that the hole had gone all way through to my mouth. On arriving back at home and later that night I was still spitting up blood and noticed that there was quite a large gap on the inside of my mouth which was around about the size of an Australian 50c coin. Over time that just closed and healed up but still left me with quite some difficulty when trying to eat and drink anything.

As I would also consider myself a decent looking young man, now having this scar and abrasion on my jaw it gave me mental and personal scars. Each day when I would get up or see myself in the mirror it was a constant reminder of what had happened and made me quite self-conscious of my appearance. I would have thoughts that people kept on looking at my face because of this scar and would my wife still love me because of this new look I was sporting? In reality it shouldn't really matter but to me it did. Even though 4-5 years later I have embraced this scar on my face and most people wouldn't realise I had been in quite a significant accident I still feel the need to have stubble and a rugged facial hair look to help hide and cover my beauty spot.

That is really quite minor compared to what happened to my mouth and jaw as a result of the impact. After numerous visits to my orthodontist and having had multiple types of x-rays done on my jaw the basic conclusion and summary to what damage had been done was quite significant. Not only had a number of my teeth been chipped and damaged, I also required root canal on the front bottom teeth as they essentially died from impact. That's nothing really compared to having your jaw fractured as well as not being able to open your mouth properly to talk, eat or chew. A typical normal functioning mouth can open 48mm up and down and laterally 11mm. Mine was at 12mm for up and down and only 3mm for lateral motion.

For the next 10-12 months, the majority of the focus was realigning my jaw so that I could open it properly to not only talk without pain but also to be able to chew food. Due to my current condition with my mouth and jaw I could no longer chew or eat food properly. For a long time, I had to have soft foods and liquids that were mashed or pureed. Talk about an inconvenience.

From the outset of the accident happening I was always going to suffer from pain, what I or the doctors didn't realise was at how bad the pain would get over time. Initially the main pain came from my mouth and jaw which is understandable considering what I had been through.

This was now also going to be the start of another big problem and major hurdle from now and for years to come afterwards. PAINKILLERS. Now there isn't anything wrong with painkillers as when you're in pain they do help relieve either some or all of that symptom. One issue though that I didn't realise at the time would happen is that by having to or depending on these painkillers that my tolerance for them would increase requiring me to take more and more of them but not necessarily helping making the pain better or go away.

Now there were a few reasons for this that I will briefly talk about as this co-aligns with part of the next bit which was the chronic pain I then started to endure.

A bit of painkiller 101 for anyone that has not had to take these silent killers often or on a regular basis: "Codeine and Opiates are highly addictive". So back to my pain, from the start I was given Panadeine Forte which is part paracetamol 500mg and codeine phosphate 30mg and comes in a box of 20 tablets. In Australia, this can't be bought over the counter. The maximum amount of codeine in a tablet that can be bought over the counter is about 13mg.

Due to the severity of my pain and accident I was prescribed to take 2 tablets four times a day. I don't know if or how many of you have taken this pill but they are reasonably strong and can make you feel pretty drowsy and dopey. So a big start to my downward spiral really started from day one as from then on I was reliant on this not so strong painkiller to what I was eventually going to be on further down the track.

Now I'm not going to go through every single drug and medication I was given or tried as I could write at least a whole chapter on that alone even possibly a book, but that's for another day and time. After a few months of having been on this drug the pain seemed to be getting worse and these pills didn't seem to be doing much. That leads to doctors putting you on new painkillers, STRONGER ones.

These new pills were now stronger than the last ones but to start with I was on a smaller dosage and weaker strength. Once again though, over the next 6 months I build up a tolerance to help alleviate the pain and by December 2012 some 10 months after the accident I'm on the strongest possible pill you can have 8 times a day before you get to the opiate family. Damn, if I was drowsy or a bit dopey on the last lot of pills imagine what I was like now and felt also. To me everything seemed to be in slow motion, my awareness diminished, concentration (well what concentration now) was no longer what it used to be and yet the pain didn't stop it was still there.

Now let's put this in perspective, over the last 10 months yes I have been in pain but the movement and re-alignment of my mouth and jaw has improved significantly. At least I now have a better range of motion and movement to be able to talk better and not have to have pureed food all the time. The only problem and issue now is that the pain is worse. How could it be worse when my mouth and jaw are getting better? Well, for one reason the pain was not so much to do with my jaw and mouth but now it came from my neck and head.

The easiest way to describe the pain I was in and some of it may be quite hard to picture but imagine someone has a hammer and is constantly tapping you on the head with it 24/7. This is no joke, it was relentless, constant and no one had the foggiest as to why and what was happening. I still have that pain to this day. Now it's by no way near the strength or the intensity of what it was 4 years ago but yes I still do suffer from this.

With this new-found pain, which we can only really describe as now Chronic Pain came another long list of challenges which I will go through shortly. With this pain came my new-found friend, well not really a friend - more of my dependent companion who quite a number of people have fallen victim to. The OPIATE family. As my pain had now reached intolerable levels I was now given OxyContin. And for your next tutorial in painkiller 101, this is one very nasty drug.

If you didn't know it is from the opium poppy family and is mainly used for people who are in significant pain or cancer sufferers. To start with I was on a fast acting form of it which means it relieves the pain sooner but for a shorter period of time which in my case didn't really help as the pain was constant and as a result without me really noticing I was taking it more often and more required than what you should. This wasn't necessarily intentional but all I wanted was relief and after a few weeks I was then moved onto the slow release version which is longer lasting, only thing was I was still on the same dosage of 4 a day even though each pill lasts for about 12 hours in theory.

Remember how earlier I explained I went from drowsy and dopey to a lot worse well now you may as well call me a zombie or someone from the walking dead, I don't think that is too high of an exaggeration either. From 2013 onwards not through any fault of my own you could have technically called me a junkie as I was dependent on an opiate and I behaved and acted as if I was high all the time. Well not so much 'if.' I Was.

One thing I should mention is that, not only having to deal with the pain side of things and the injury itself, but not long after the initial accident I would suffer from flashbacks of the incident or other types of instances that related to pain. I would soon find out that this is commonly called Post Traumatic Stress Disorder (PTSD) and for quite a long time I would have episodes during the middle of the night which would wake me up and in turn my wife. The really bad cases I can still remember would have me rolling around vigorously in my bed while asleep, along with screaming and in a panic.

On one occasion I managed to cause bruises on my wife, mainly due to the kicking or flailing arms while rolling around, and also knock over my bedside table and everything on it. Things were broken or smashed on numerous occasions. That was only one example of what would happen and there were many other things that would happen to me also but we don't really need to go into all of them.

With all these things that were going on in my life and working towards the deterioration of my health and wellbeing did the depression start to kick in. Life was tough, I had gone from being an active outgoing person who had so much to offer and give in society to someone who was in pain, down in confidence, couldn't work, doped up and just in general was really struggling. I knew that this would probably enter the fray at some stage once the accident had happened, but I didn't really know how quickly it would take to set in - or how bad it would be.

What you have to understand with depression is that if you're the person who is suffering from it, it's not always the easiest to admit or detect that you are in that sort of rut or frame of mind as such. On the other side of the equation you have your friends, family, and my case wife also that could see the rise and fall of their loved one and the effects it had on our relationships. Looking back at it now this really is tough for all who are involved and have to deal with people that have or suffer from depression.

The biggest and best piece of advice I can suggest and say to you from the family/friend/partner side of things is don't try to understand or even determine what we are going through. Because if you've never been through it you just won't get it. Even though you only have the best intentions for us and want to help in every possible way, we're not looking for advice. What we want is for someone just to sit and listen and be there for us. Is it a challenge? Of course it is, as there will be days or hours in the day that we are doing fine and then next minute we're not, we are struggling just to keep our eyes open and have no motivation to do anything.

The worst thing that a person could say to me is: 'just get up and do something, snap out of it.' It doesn't really work like that. In the next section I'll share with you certain things that I adopted that ultimately helped me in time. For me though it did take quite a substantial amount of time.

Unfortunately, due to my worsening condition from other symptoms and injuries that were appearing over time due to the damage that stemmed from the pressure of my neck, spine and head which was causing all this other severe chronic pain as well as the mood swings from my depression and pain medication that it caused the breakdown of my relationship with my wife and ultimately led to her leaving me.

Kick a man while he's down right and yes I have seen this happen on multiple occasions, though to her defense she had stuck around for two years of my suffering. We aren't here to talk about whether she should have stayed by my side and been there through sickness and health, till death do us part. She did what she needed to do and felt was best for her.

For me this was a massive kick in the teeth as not only was I struggling with the day to day life struggles, the pain medication, all the trips to doctors and specialists on a weekly basis for my rehab along with having to worry about the future court case and legal action that just seemed to go on and on even though the matter was pretty clear cut and simple. These things aren't as straight forward and as simple as one would think but there was also financial stress because of the medical bills and expenses that were all out of pocket until the legal matter was resolved. This wouldn't finally take place until over 3 years after the accident actually happening.

Life for me was just becoming too much to handle with all this stress in my life, it wasn't just one thing but a culmination of 4 or more things that compounded to it. Effectively 2 years after the actual accident on February 25th 2014 life for me just became too difficult. What I failed to mention earlier was that with all the things that I was going through on top of that I wouldn't get much sleep either mainly due to the pain. It still happens to me now but on average I would only get 2-3 hours of sleep a night if I was lucky. It just takes a toll on your body and mental state.

On this day in February a few things happened which I'm not going to go into but were contributing factors towards where my mind was heading. This added to the fact that I hadn't really had any sleep for 2-3 days, so was pretty exhausted. I was extremely upset and I couldn't see an end to my situation or anything positive coming from my life.

At that point and this was a spur of the moment thing as I had never in the past felt like self-harming myself. I had just had enough. At this point I was just in full meltdown mode, I was sorry for all the pain and suffering I had caused to others during these last few years. How my mood and actions had ultimately affected my ex-wife, her family as well as my own family and friends. I felt like that they were better off without me in this world. I didn't think of the consequences it would have or cause to them nor how they would feel or handle this action I was about to do.

I don't feel it was selfish it was just how I was feeling and felt at that point in time. I was tired, sore and alone in life. Without any hesitation I crushed a copious amount of my painkillers and sleeping pills. To be honest with you, there was enough there to sink a battleship. The pile was huge and I just snorted it in one go as that is the quickest way to get it into your system without having to swallow a whole lot of pills. Before I ingested the substances I said or had a message for God. I said "God I'm tired and I'm sorry, either I'm going to have a good sleep or a long sleep. I'll leave that decision up to you." I then proceeded to send my ex and two best friends a message with the words "I'm Sorry" and headed to bed for a lie down. I had no idea what would or was going to happen next.

Fortunately, my ex took the message with a serious note of concern even though we weren't together anymore and notified my father. What my father and family experienced next no parent should ever have to witness or go through but seeing his son lie there motionless on the bed, not moving, and not knowing if he's going to wake up could be quite distressing as one would imagine. I ended up in ICU for 3 days and am very lucky and fortunate to still be alive.

Things That Helped Me Get Through Certain Parts

It wasn't just the attempted suicide that was the wakeup call I needed. There were a number of things that I needed to work on and change in my life. One thing I did know was that I wanted to get off these pills and I wanted a better life than what I was currently living. Something needed to change but I knew it had to start with me.

I couldn't be reliant on others to do it for me. It was really at that point I told my doctor that I was going to wean myself off the pills and could she help keep me accountable as this part I did need help and encouragement with to get me through it. At this point I was on over 100mg or equivalent to 12-16 10mg of OxyContin pills a day.

One thing I have always been good at throughout my life is if I set my mind to something, I do it. I'm quite a determined and goal focused person who has competed in sport at a high level, so I know what it takes to succeed and get through challenging times. This is no different.

Between the pain specialist, doctor, and myself we worked on a plan and strategy to come off a certain amount of these pills each month and work towards the goal of being on the least number of pills possible that I could manage.

It's amazing what the mind and body can do when you have something you really want to achieve.

I've always had faith and hope that I would get through this turmoil even though I was told by numerous doctors and specialists that I would be in pain for the rest of my life and that they didn't know if my situation would get better or worse. I never accepted that prognosis and I'm glad I didn't. I didn't know then how I was going to get through it all. But I knew deep within myself was that I would get through it.

Now what you must understand and realise is that from birth I was brought up by Catholic parents and grandparents as well as schooling and friends. It is something that I respected and followed for most my life. Along the way, I stopped being the regular church-goer but I have never stopped having faith or hope even when times got tough. Along the way even though I wasn't so prevalent to it and have only really found out recently, is that people have always been looking out for me by either praying or just watching out for me. So, for me personally God has had a big impact on my life, not by just resolving and making the situation go away but by helping me get through the tough times. For all that I have experienced and endured it has made me such a better person. It has taught me how to ask and to forgive others, just like the personal trainer who dropped the weight on my face. To not judge others or their circumstances, to live in peace, joy and to love one another and that there's no point being bitter or hold resentment against others for what I have been and had being going through. I realise that now. The past is the past and is not the future or my future.

Over a 10-month period roughly from Feb to Dec 2015 I managed to go from 16 pills a day to 3-4 which is a great achievement. It took a lot of perseverance, commitment as well as discipline not to take more than I had to even if the pain was unbearable. As I was still unable to work properly and didn't have employment I knew I had to keep myself busy or occupied. It was a gradual process but I started walking again. To begin with I was only able to manage 15 minutes at a time. I would do this once a day and then build that up to twice.

Then I could do 30 minutes at a time, then twice a day and so on. Along with that I started to want to get back into other hobbies that I loved but had neglected or just didn't have the motivation to do. For me one of those things is cooking, for you it could be drawing, reading, painting. Whatever it is all you need to do is make a start, even if it's for a few minutes and then slowly work your way into doing it as often as you need or want to do.

Something else that helped me was the night before I would write a list of things that I needed to get done for the day and week, it would generally entail about 5-10 things on it. As long as I ticked off at least one of those items on my list of things to do then I considered it making progress. If I did 2 or more then that was just a bonus and by doing this on a daily and weekly basis I started to get myself back into routine of getting what needed to be done rather than just think about it in my head and then not do it. I still do this routine today and I know the days when I don't do this, they tend to be my least productive days.

I did also benefit from utilising other resources in early 2016 which has not only helped me with overcoming my depression but in also coming off all my medication which included anti-inflammatories, sleeping pills, anti-depressants, and OxyContin for the pain. On April 25th of 2016 I stopped taking all these pharmaceutical drugs and now 7 months on I feel like a new person with no need or desire to touch or want to go back on to them at all.

The one resource that helped me in coming off the prescription drugs was a book I was given to read from a very close personal friend who has been looking and watching over me for a very long time and is also big part of why I am still here and have become the person I am today. I owe that person everything I have and glad that she has always been there for me even if we do live in different countries.

The book that she gave me is called "Chasing the Dragon" by Jackie Pullinger. I won't go into great detail into what it's about but briefly the story revolves around an English lady who is a missionary that heads to Hong Kong in the 1960-70's. It wasn't just Hong Kong that she went to but the infamous walled city which in the 1960s was not policed and consequently had become one of the world's largest opium producing centres, run by Chinese criminal Triad gangs. Later she established a youth club that helped the drug addicts and street sleepers inside the walled city.

The 2nd book that I read which helped me get through and help me overcome my depression was "Healthy Thinking, How to Turn Life's Lemons into Lemonade" by Dr Tom Mulholland. What this book did for me was help give me a massive reality check but also provide me with tools and information that I could use on a daily basis with initially coping with the depression and then eventually getting through it. It doesn't happen overnight but with persistence and perseverance it did happen.

These are just a couple of things that helped me along the way with my recovery. There are many more that I am also grateful for and those will come out in time when I decide to write the extended version of this story.

Where I'm at now and my commitment to helping others with their personal struggles

One of the main positives of the accident is that it made me realise that I need to do what I am good at, what I love and what I am passionate about. For me this involves working with property. Since I was 10 years old I have been involved in renovations and purchasing property. This is either for myself or with my father. I studied it at University and up until the accident had only been doing it for ourselves as a hobby. It is something that can help you make decent money.

And it can set you up for life - whether it be for your own personal lifestyle, retirement or just so you are able to spend more time with your kids and family. I now teach, educate, and speak to people about how they can get into the property market if they haven't already done so and how they can also grow their current property portfolio in order to free up time for the things they actually want to do in life. I've done this in multiple countries and will continue to do so in the future.

Secondly, and part of the reason I chose to write this chapter, was to share my story and to help others. I knew I had a purpose. Even though I have suffered and have been through quite a bit, I have managed to get through it. Hopefully my story will give you hope that, no matter what you're going through, someone else has been there and gone through it. You may suffer from depression, trauma, PTSD, chronic pain, injury, addictions, attempted suicide, or the like. The one thing you can take strength from is the fact that I have been there and I have prevailed. "If I Can, You Can".

Anjay Zazulak

About The Author

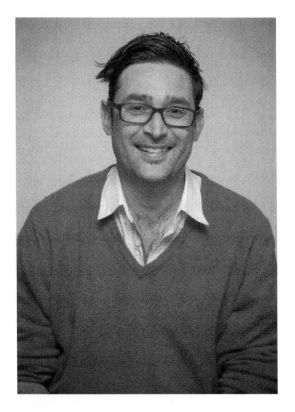

Anjay Zazulak – Property Buyer/Speaker/Mentor/Co-Author

What I Do
I assist buyers to find the right property at the right price by putting an end to the frustrations of the buying process! Whether you're looking to purchase your Principal Place of Residence (PPOR) or Investment Property(s), Our Buyers Agent services include all aspects of searching out the right property and checking that it suits your criteria.

What I have found over the years and the questions I so often get asked is:

- Where to start and what to buy
- Homeowners tend to look in a 5-10km radius of where they live or where they grew up
- They think that property is not necessarily affordable for them which isn't always the case
- People are hesitant to purchase or invest as they think it will impact their lifestyle
- Are afraid of the risks and horror stories they so often hear as well as all the clutter that is provided by the media and lack of knowledge and education provided

Who I Serve
Those who are time poor, are frustrated with the buying process or just have no idea on where to start or what to buy. I've been teaching and helping people from the Planning stage right through to Settlement in securing that next purchase.

How I Do It
I empower you to feel confident in your purchase and we provide professional support services to assist you every step of the way. We'll dispel many of the myths surrounding real estate and show you just how easy and rewarding purchasing your next property can be.

Who I Work With
Those people who are looking to purchase their next property whether it's for them to live in or as an investment for your personal portfolio.

My Style
Highly engaging, dynamic, honest, up front and fun... I make the confusing world of buying property easy to understand and enjoyable again.

Anjay gets his biggest kick from sharing his knowledge and expertise with his clients, facilitating their realisations that property is within their reach. He's always amazed that it takes only a little bit of action to get someone started.

Having purchased over 30 properties in 3 different countries, including New Zealand, Australia and Japan, Anjay has the experience to help people, even in different countries to get their start in property and avoid the pitfalls and mistakes common to investors.

To find out more or to talk to Anjay Zazulak about his take on property investing or men's/mental health:

Email: ajzazulak@gmail.com
LinkedIn: au.linkedin.com/in/anjayzazulak

Becoming Myself

Four and a half years ago Lisa's life changed dramatically, and forever. Now, still in her forties and a survivor of brain haemorrhage and a stroke, her future looks very different from the one she'd imagined. Here is her story…

Early in January 2011 I woke after a good night's sleep with a mild headache. I roused my husband Russell and asked for a tablet, before the pain became excruciatingly severe and I felt as if I was about to die. Minutes later the paramedics arrived as I threw up over the carpet, I was moved onto a stretcher and taken downstairs to the ambulance. I still clearly remember my daughters' confused little faces framed between the bars of the banister watching as I was carried out of the house. Was I being taken out of their lives too?

I had suffered a severe type of sub-arachnoid haemorrhage (a bleeding in the brain), which I was very lucky to survive. (only 2% of patients who experience brain aneurysm survive this After being taken to the local accident and emergency unit I was in a coma, on life support for several weeks and only learned long afterwards of all the intervention that had taken place to save my life. I had been so close to death or alternatively, to a persistent vegetative state, that my husband was advised to bring our daughters into the hospital to witness it for themselves to prepare them for the likely unhappy ending. As well as being put on a life support machine, a section of my skull was removed to accommodate my swollen brain.

At one stage during medical intervention I suffered a second bleed and a stroke, and this has left me totally paralysed on my left side. When I returned to the conscious world., the tracheotomy meant that I could still not eat, drink or talk. I did not know for many months that my husband had been warned by doctors that I might have remained in a permanent vegetative state forever. I still could not move my left side, eat, drink, or speak, or see properly.

At first it was a challenge to stay positive. Every five minutes I would set myself challenges to accomplish minor things that were no longer easy, such as could I ring my bell and ask for a bed pan in time to do the right thing in the right place? I had lost my swallow reflex and this meant I could neither eat nor drink or even swallow my own saliva, which left me permanently hungry, thirsty, drooling and feeling as if I had gone a bit mad. I felt totally degraded. When the greatest accomplishment in a day is the correct use of a bed pan, you know that you've sunk pretty low. I was surprised by the lack of knowledge amongst the medics about my swallowing problem. I was treated like a recalcitrant schoolchild who was deliberately choosing not to swallow even when Russell kindly brought in homemade food to stimulate a response. But it was impossible for me to swallow or taste it. I hated the stroke ward and its elderly patients and their heart-rending cries for help. I felt powerless to help them. The only thing I could do was to ring my call bell for attention and redirect the nurse to the distressed lady, a trick I had learned from a now-friend called Vera, who used to help me out when I couldn't reach mine.

It's a humbling feeling to be totally reliant on your call bell to communicate.   Stripped of any independent agency to do anything, although I did offer to help a very old lady who may have had dementia . She wanted her hand held all day but the nurses couldn't sit with her. I asked them to wheel my bed next to hers so that I could hold her hand to give her some comfort . It helped me too, by making me feel useful and needed again

Around this time the grief began: I was acutely missing Russell and the girls. I was inconsolable and cried all day long missing my family and also, perhaps, myself as I was no longer the same person. What I wanted most of all was to get back to my life as a busy mum and my part-time marketing job with a local Kent theatre. All that seemed to have been taken away from me. I was prescribed anti-depressants, and these put me into a permanent state of drowsiness. Enveloped in inescapable fatigue I barely felt any connection with the real world anymore and on one memorable occasion I could not open my eyes or talk properly to a dear friend who'd travelled for hours from Somerset to visit me in Kent.

I received many cards and letters from friends, relations and former colleagues, which I kept in a large box on the windowsill in my room near my bed. I would spend hours staring at that box and mulling over its contents – it gave me strength to think positively and to continue trying to get better. If so many people wanted me to 'get well soon', then surely I must! At this stage I was reminding myself daily of my primary school motto: "I am I can I ought I will. " It helped me to draw on the strength developed from childhood , so that I knew I would survive and get better.

Finally, after thirteen months in various hospitals and a couple of brief home visits to finalise my in-home care package, I was discharged in time for Christmas. It was a fantastic feeling. I had truly believed that I was going to miss Christmas with my family completely. But no, my sister was waiting to greet me at home with the girls, balloons and a fabulous welcome home cake made by my elder daughter. But it was only now, returning home, that I became truly aware of the loss that had occurred in the intervening months: my daughters were now 8 and 10. They had grown up and I had missed the small, daily changes that occur for any growing child. I felt odd, too. Although I'd longed to be here for more than a year I could no longer do things I'd previously taken for granted. I couldn't potter around the kitchen or go upstairs to our bedroom or to the girls' bedrooms to check on them, even though they no longer required a bedtime story from me.

Initially, I slept downstairs in a bed provided by the hospital and needed a hoist and two people to lift me to sit in my wheelchair. This, and the fact that I was still being peg fed via a tube directly to my stomach because of my swallowing difficulties and subsequent weight loss, made it obvious to the girls that, while I was home at last, I was still a patient. And because I could not yet fall asleep comfortably I kept the radio on all night to stop my thoughts from wandering back to the hospital ward.

Shortly afterwards I met my physiotherapist, Jo, whose no-nonsense manner was literally a life-saver. We began an exercise regime with the dual goals of walking again and managing the stairs as I was determined not to ruin the character and layout of our house by having a lift installed. I discovered how resilient and single minded I could be. The first time that Jo stood me up again it was quite frightening after such a long time spent horizontally, but it gave me a taste for what might be possible. Although there were no steps yet, I knew my long journey would start with standing and eventually a single step.

My package of hospital care was transferred to one of home care, allowing Tiia to move in as my full-time, live-in carer. While we were lucky to have the space to accommodate her, it was a major adjustment for the rest of the family. Tiia was very committed. And sensitive. She brought stability to all of us, encouraging me to do my exercises, supporting Russell and the girls, and helping me to become involved in family life again. As I once again learnt how be a mother, I felt cheated by life and angry too. The girls' tastes and eating habits had changed and I relished choosing menus for them, although it took some time for me to catch up with the new evening routine where they no longer had a separate tea, bath and bedtime story, preferring instead to have supper with us, and afterwards showering themselves before choosing their own night reading. Where had my little girls gone?

Once I had settled in and getting through each day no longer seemed a small miracle. During this period I had been working relentlessly with my carers I learnt to bear weight on my legs again and built my upper body strength until I was finally able to sit unsupported. I began to think about living again. I developed my own idiosyncratic method and eventually I got up those stairs and now sleep in my own bedroom every night and use my own bathroom which still feels like a treat each day and realised how much of myself had been a mother (which, of course, I still am). But the girls had changed and so had I. It was time to reinvent myself: but what could I do and what did I want to do? I was fortunate to have retained my bank of knowledge and experience – the damage to my brain had affected the part that deals with sight (leaving me partially sighted unable to read – and I felt a strong need to work again. I wanted to use the skills I still had and achieve something worthwhile, so I jumped at the opportunity to assist with marketing projects in the fund raising department of a the Hospice in the Weald offering end of life care to cancer sufferers and the elderly.

Returning to work in a voluntary capacity made sense as I was still uncertain about my limitations and my stamina was building slowly. As I learnt to manage daily life with post-stroke fatigue I was allocated a desk and it felt good to be back in the hustle and bustle of an office again, although my sight deficiency and brain damage made it difficult to use a computer screen or deal with basic number sequencing. But I have been slowly developing coping strategies. I remain determined to show the girls that it is possible for women to work even when there are significant obstacles to overcome. Imagination, flexibility and self-belief, resourcefulness and resilience can make the impossible seem possible again. I single-mindedly focussed on what I could do and stopped thinking about what I couldn't do or had missed out on.

My new mantra became: "it's not about who I used to be but about who I will become now". I adjusted myself to the enforced inactivity which comes with hemi-paralysis and decided to use the additional time spent at home to my advantage, by updating my professional skills to be current in an online world dominated by social networking. I studied an online course with the Hubspot Academy and learnt my way around Twitter and Facebook, both of which I had despised before my stroke (probably due to my lack of knowledge about how they work). I also used the time to follow an online course run by Janet Murray (Soulful PR). I found the digital marketing course interesting. The exam was far harder than I had overconfidently expected. After a few attempts I was successful and was awarded my certificate in inbound marketing.

Simultaneously I had become involved with a local arts project. Rusthall Community Arts is a creative community engagement project which strives to inspire the community through the arts. I have met stimulating, like-minded people who, like me, value the nourishing contribution which the arts can make. Writing, music, visual arts, performance, and craft can bring people together and improve mental health by providing an outlet for self-expression. I discovered that my life-long love of poetry needed to be further fulfilled by writing my own material, two examples of which I have included at the end of this chapter.

I currently remain an unpublished poet but who knows? On behalf of the festival activity I began to regularly attend a local networking coffee morning known as twitter group. Here I met local business men and pitched myself to them in the hope of securing paid work. I recognise that this may seem pushy but I actually felt happier trying to convince someone to take me on face to face since I was not hiding my limitations. They could see that I was paralysed and struggled with my vision. After a few months good fortune finally came my way when I met an ambitious American who was setting up a company in the field of advertising and technology. We struck up a rapport. He needed some extra assistance inexpensively and I needed a job without pressure or responsibility. We reached a mutually beneficial arrangement and I received a contract to work 8 hours per week as his Web Content Manager. I finally felt a little of my self-respect returning.

That was in April 2016, more than five years after my haemorrhage. At that time I continued to work hard with my new , physiotherapist , David, in the pool doing hydrotherapy I had previously tried hydrotherapy at the hospital with disappointing results. It was thanks to the encouragement of a new friend whom I met at Twitter group that I was given the push to try again this time with David at Burrswood until he felt that I was ready to try walking on land again (without the support of a stick). Against the backdrop of the divisive campaigning around the Brexit Referendum I mentally prepared myself for those first steps. On June 23rd 2016, I took my first unsupported steps I still had no feeling whatsoever in my left leg or foot So did not know when my left foot reached the ground but relied on my strength of mind to believe that I would not fall if I lifted my right foot up to take a step and I did it I walked a few steps with no stick for support my carer Tiia was still with me and she filmed these precious first steps on my phone It was not yet fluid walking but it is a start from which I intend to improve until I reach my personal goal of walking and dancing at my fiftieth birthday next year .In November we heard that Rusthall Festival had won a prize in our local Heart of the Community Awards ,sponsored by AXAPPP I attended the ceremony and was pushed up to receive the award from the mayor and gave an off the cuff thank you speech I felt so proud for my colleagues, the project and for myself for being a part of it and being alive too . There really is a joy and thrill to be found in living when you've been so close to losing it all

I had this feeling when my husband and I made a recent trip to Paris last year. This was a trip which we had promised ourselves and planned during those dark hospital days by train. Sitting in a rooftop bar overlooking the city and the Eiffel Tower as we sipped champagne, I felt very alive, if a little not restricted by my wheelchair. Although even this had unexpected benefits, such as being fast-tracked to the front of the queue at the Louvre and to see the Mona Lisa by a sympathetic attendant. Yes, I wish I could wander around the gallery and walk the banks of the Seine, but this is my new kind of normal now and it's not all bad. I am continuing to achieve things each day

I took my first steps without the aid of a stick on June 23rd 2016, hereafter known not only as Independence Day (Brexit) but also as Independent walking day for me . Albeit this achievement has only taken place in physiotherapy so far, under the watchful care of my current physio David. But I now know that I can do it and that one day I will walk unaided again.

So what has seen me through all of this? I would not have got here without a number of key factors:

Family and friends have provided constant support and encouragement to me through some dark days. My sisters and my parents have accepted me as I am throughout my journey. My husband has shown remarkable strength, maintaining our home life for our daughters without the wife he married. There's been rather more of the "in sickness" than either of us anticipated. My daughters will always be the source of much of my strength I want to be the mother that they deserve.

FAITH I found that I have a far deeper Catholic faith than I knew beforehand the bread of life seemed to literally help me to return to life . I have been humbled by the dedication shown by Eucharistic ministers who have visited me consistently at home and in hospital to offer me communion and prayers. I now strongly believe in the power of prayer to make a difference. I feel blessed that I have had the opportunity to discover this for myself.

Creativity: my own creativity has proven to be of much greater importance to me than in the past.

Community: I have discovered the supportive value which is offered by community. Both real and virtual. My involvement in the community project in Rusthall has been life affirming , the Catholic Church is all about community and participation. I have been enormously supported , emotionally by a group of people which I have only encountered online thanks to the charity for younger stroke survivors, Different Strokes. Through this I communicate with fellow stroke survivors through a moderated Facebook group which has given me access to a group of people that can empathise with my predicaments.

They may be strangers in the real world but in the virtual world they have genuinely become my friends as individuals who are prepared to give and receive support when needed. My husband has, of course, seen what I've gone through but he can never know what it has been like as well as someone who has experienced a similar journey . We are all active in the group busy getting on with our lives. I like to refer to us as "livers" rather than survivors.

We do so much more than survive and can rely on each other we help to make each other stronger which I have tried to capture in a poem:

Two Skeletons

I've got two skeletons,

I'm stronger than I knew ,

And so are you

There's 270 bones at birth and to give strength, mobility and

protection

If I Can, You Can

I had a strong start

one was enough for me

then

I was strong, active and safe

When I needed it I found my second ,

The fusion of faith, friends, family, creativity, love

which made me even stronger

kept me active, safe, happy, alive, moving forward

Yours won't be like mine

but it's there

but keep it quiet

SCULPTED

I

HAVE BEEN SCULPTED

CHIP, followed by blow and blow

Before my material was concealed

My true form is now defined

WHEN the stroke hit me I did not crack

I tried hard not to look back

It is the material with which you start that matters most

The material took shape and was refined

A new me

Confusing for those who thought they knew me

Time to start again a new encounter

Who knew life is a sculptor?

So what has seen me through all of this? I would not have got here without a number of key factors:

CARERS: I have been very fortunate to have benefited from the support and friendship of a few dedicated live-in carers without whom I would not have made my progress while maintaining family life too. Thank you so much Tiia, Wendy, Sharon and Fiona and Agnes and Christianne who have held us all together. Each one has developed an intimate understanding of my needs.

Putting my story onto paper has been far harder than I expected. Now that I have to adapt to the limitation of my partial sight and my brain damage, which has left me unable to read easily, to punctuate correctly, and to plan effectively. I owe a debt of gratitude to my husband and a friend for helping to make this chapter a reality.

So if someone who faced the prognosis of a persistent vegetative state can get published in a book aptly named "If I can you can" then imagine what else might be possible if you fire your imagination.

Lisa Beaumont

About The Author

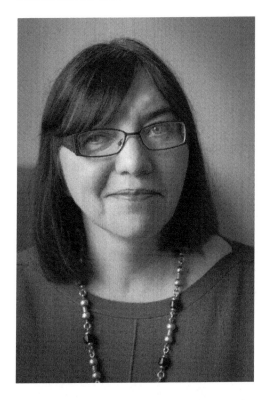

Lisa Beaumont is a mother, wife, stroke survivor, Communications Director for Rusthall Community Arts, poet, marketing practitioner and social media fan. Radio4 addict and friend She is guided by her favourite quotation: "And the end of all our exploring will be to arrive where we started and know the place for the first time" (TS Eliot, Little Gidding).

If I Can, You Can

www.rusthallcommunityarts.org.uk

Twitter @ArtRusthall

@thebeaumonts1

Facebook: Rusthall Community Arts

Self-Belief And Hard Work Really Do Matter

My name is Luke and I am a 30 year old entrepreneur from Birmingham. I own a few small to medium sized business that all turn a healthy profit year on year, which gives me the financial freedom to really maximize life. But believe me it has not been a straight forward journey and I am a very different person today from who I was not that long ago.

Underachiever

Growing up I had extremely supportive parents who gave me every chance in life to be successful - whether that be from an academic perspective, a sporting one or any other one for that matter. Unfortunately at the time I was like most teenagers; ungrateful, selfish and took their help and support for granted. I expected them to take me to my football matches plus training four times per week and my cross-country races, without really considering the impact I was having on their life. You could say I was selfish, but I like to think of it as 'unaware' or that I was very egocentric in my ways at that age.

Lack Of Focus

After stumbling through my GCSEs - and I do mean stumbling - achieving far lower than I know I was capable of, followed by disappointing A-levels, which in truth I only went into as I did not know what else to do with myself, life was ticking by without any real goals, purpose or aspirations. I even tried to go to university, paid for again by my parents. In this I, again, formulated a pattern of disappointment by dropping out, not once, but three times! The third time I did genuinely give it a good go and was getting very good feedback from tutors and obtaining very high marks on my assignments. But unfortunately I did have a problem with going out far too much and after a sticky break up with my girlfriend at the time, I soon fell behind on my assignments and, back then, quitting was easy for me when things got tough.

This coupled with my older brother's success after he graduated from Cambridge with a first class honors degree and a masters in engineering, showed really the gulf in attitude between the two of us. I was low, very low. Sometimes I would cry at night until I fell asleep as I felt like my life was just pointless. I had not achieved anything and nothing seemed to be on the horizon for me to look forward to, from a work perspective or a relationship one and it was hard to watch friends and family achieving things around me. I used play down their success stories in my own mind to make myself feel better and that everyone's life is terminal anyway, so why bother.

I then worked in a few low paid jobs that got me by and stayed with LA fitness as a sales advisor for several years, which I enjoyed and was very good at, more naturally than hard work. I was and still am a people's person, so sales was a natural position for me. The role was a very basic sales role though and was not challenging for me, but I loved going the gym and saw it as a possible career for me. I still had the same old problems though; lack of drive to succeed, prioritizing going out over work and, some days, I just did not turn up as I simply did not feel like it. I had an awful manager at the time, which did not help matters.

When management roles presented themselves, I was

subsequently overlooked. I used to blame LA Fitness for not giving me a chance at management, but in reality I was not working hard enough, was not ready for the role or making myself the obvious candidate. After the last disappointment, I went to a doctor as I was suffering from depression at the age of 23. That in its own right is depressing. I kept thinking to myself, "I could do this job with my eyes closed. Why are they choosing someone else over me? How is that guy in charge when I'm not?" I genuinely could not understand it and I started to become arrogant, which seems ironic since I really had nothing to be arrogant about. I think it was a defence mechanism and I started blaming the system for my failures and the reason why I did not have to try or dedicate myself to anything. I clearly remember saying several times "I don't need to justify my ability, people should recognise it". I now know how ridiculous this statement sounds.

Did I contemplate suicide at one point? Yes! Honestly though, I never would have done it. That takes guts. At this point in my heart of hearts I considered myself a loser and someone who justified failure with excuses. We all fail, I do it at least once per week, but nowadays I try and I know I try harder than everybody else. This does not mean that the result will be better but the effort is always 100%. I work relentlessly towards my goals and I'm the first to arrive and last to leave, not just in our office, but in the entire building complex where our head office is situated. I even set the security alarms off four times, which can only be done if someone is occupying the office past 1am.

Inspiration

The moment I truly realised the situation I was in came in the form of a few small events. I remember saying to my work colleague who was performing the same role as me at LA Fitness "Nothing is going right for me, I am seriously fed up, are you not fed up getting talked down to by a manger that both of us are more capable than?" She turned to me and said "No! " She then stood up and wrote down on the white board a label of categories from relationship, family, money, job satisfaction and a few others and asked me to rate each one out of ten with ten being the most satisfied and one of course being the least. She then asked me to rate where I think they should be at this stage of my life. After I completed it, I stood back and realised work was the lowest at a two and I thought it should be at least an eight. That was the first time I actually evaluated the cause and the reason why I was unhappy.

Within a few days my dad, who was a vice principal at a school and head of discipline there, said to me "you remind me son of one of the students I have just expelled. He told me he likes to do well, but he doesn't want to do well". At first I was confused, as both ideas initially seemed like the same thing. Actually the reality is very different. What he meant was that wanting is where you work for something and that you make the end goal happen and liking is where you hope something will happen.

After explaining this he said "honestly, if you are unhappy, what have you done to rectify the situation, what action have you taken?" I could not answer him as the answer was absolutely nothing and he was right. People talk about motivation and inspiration to change their habits and this was mine. I was fed up and in truth I was getting bored of being fed up. It was time to do something about it and be accountable for myself.

I was the reason why I did not get the LA Fitness role and looking back now I wouldn't even have interviewed me, let alone hire me. I did not do well at my GCSEs and A-Levels, as I did not deserve to do well. If it was not for my parents, and being extremely lucky in having a very helpful and supportive family, who knows where I would be right now. One problem though; I needed a plan and somewhere to direct my new found drive.

The Plan

I loved watching business based programmes, the likes of Dragons Den and the apprentice when it first came out. Like everybody else I used to scream at the television thinking that something was glaringly obvious that they had missed in their business plan or that their service lacked a key fundamental to make it thrive. I had always thought how amazing it would be to run my own business and that, if I were working for myself. I would give it my absolute everything to make it a success

It was decided. I was going to start my own gym! One problem, I had no assets, no house, no car and I was 24 with no real career to speak of. This time I did not get upset and give up like every time before. But the new found motivation that I had said, Ok, how can I overcome this? The thought of owning my own gym (although it felt a million miles away) was always fresh in my mind.

I spoke with the bank and they politely told me I was not investable. This was at the time when banks handed business loans out like confetti at a wedding and I still could not get a loan. I then thought to myself how can I get the capital to start this business? It then dawned on me that my brother had cleared his university debts playing poker online and I wondered if I could do the same?

Finding A Goal Changed My Life!

I started playing for fake money for practice but soon realised this does not actually help at all as poker only works If there is value attached to bets. So I started playing for tiny amounts of real cash online, money I could afford to lose, like £2 here and there.

I was getting hooked, but it was fun too. But I wanted it to be more than fun, I needed to get better and quick if I wanted to start opening my own business.

My brother used to make thousands of dollars online when he was doing it.

I started reading book after book and watching hours of strategy videos in my spare time as well as playing more and more. Within months I was now playing and consistently winning at levels where I could even stop work if I wanted to. Every day I would come straight home from work, login online and start playing until bedtime and then repeat this process all week. I felt like my life had purpose and that at last I had a goal and an entity that I enjoyed to focus my attention on. Although progress was slow, I felt happier as I knew I was building towards something for the first time and other aspects of my life improved through this focus. Within eighteen months I got my driving license, bought a house, changed my job with a much healthier salary and had virtually stopped drinking. For the first time I was working hard at something that I wanted to achieve, all with owning a gym in mind at the end of it. I was starting to acknowledge that it was hard work, drive and having a goal that allowed me to achieve this. I stopped blaming everybody else and did the work-required to achieve something.

The Job That Inspired The Launch Of My First Business

After a while poker was getting very taxing. It is very ant-social and you had to play every evening and on your weekends as that is where the action is. It also became very stressful the higher I played and I lost the kick of getting a win as I expected to win. And when runs of bad luck occur, it would make me feel low, which, as a poker player, you have to just accept, shrug your shoulders and move on to the next hand. The decision to stop playing was a calculated one and unlike everything else I have ever stopped in the past was due to a good work life balance and not because I could not hack it anymore. I was still very determined to start my own gym and had even written a business plan and visited a couple of potential sites that I thought would be great areas to start a business.

At this point work at my new job was going really well. I was promoted to National Sales Manager for the fitness education company that I was working for. I was running my own team and was even named employee of the year. This was a really proud moment for me and I couldn't wait to share it with my parents. They had supported me continuously despite all the disappointments and they were talking about me with high esteem to their friends. The feeling of satisfaction that gave me was immense. I knew I was going places and in truth in did not matter anymore if I got there or not, just that I was at least trying to.

As I was getting more involved with senior managerial decisions I started to notice some very unethical behavior in the organisation. This was especially so in relation to the treatment of particular staff members. The behaviour also included the manner in which they dealt with complaints and lacked a desire to even consider improving their customer service. Every time I raised a concern about the value we were giving the students or an issue regarding complaints they were handled really abruptly and I was shut down for even making suggestions. Clear cases of criminal activity that I will not mention for legal reasons were staring me in the face and this created a huge moral dilemma for me. I had the promotion that I actually deserved but it was getting embarrassing to be a part of the organization. After a sit down with my parents (again), they asked: "Do you think you could do something like that better?" Of course, that is it! I knew I could do this better and without having to compromise my own ethics.

Always Take Action

I had savings aplenty now and, although I still wanted to own a gym, I saw this as an excellent avenue to help me reach my goal. I felt mentally ready to be able to do this. I had lost the sense of doubt that I used to have about myself that I used to mask with arrogance. But I knew I needed a business partner who was teaching qualified to actually get the business functioning. The new determined me approached Steph who was working as a freelance tutor for the same company but I knew she had her own business on the side, a private personal training studio. We are a similar age and she was a qualified tutor. I sent her an email highlighting my ambitions and that I wanted her to be my business partner. I believed I had established myself within that company as a good quality member of staff and Steph and I had met once before and had a good conversation about the state of the industry.

After a couple of discussions on the phone we arranged to meet in Liverpool to discuss our USP (Unique Selling Point) and what we thought the company we worked for lacked and where the gap in the market was. Before long we had a strategy of attack, a unique selling point; We would own our own venues and run our courses out of our own facilities while only using active personal trainers as our student's mentors. However there was one problem: Steph lived in Liverpool and I lived in Birmingham. I say this was a problem, but now not a lot was a problem for me, I was ready, happy and extremely motivated.

I Packed Up & Left

Without a second thought I handed in my notice with my current employers. I set-up a business account, which I deposited my life savings in, and moved to Liverpool. It was literally as quick as that and Origym was born.

I sold my house and, after one month to raise funds, I sold my car to pay for things like our website as well as our initial marketing plan. I also paid for all of the approvals that are required by the governing body to verify that our training is suitable for purpose. Using Steph's existing facility to act as our head office we went all guns blazing, working between 80 and 100 hours per week, while not taking one penny in salary for the first eight months. I now had no car, no house and no money. But I did the same white board test for myself as I did two years earlier. And I gave both job and life satisfaction a nine out of ten. It did not matter that I had no car, no house or no money. I was formulating a career that I was proud of.

Things were going well. Our bank balance was looking healthy, we had built up our social media following, our brand was looking on point and the freedom of being my own boss felt amazing.

Rising To The Challenge

Steph was a great teacher and I like to feel that I was a good at sales. So we had most bases covered that our business would require. However there were certain areas of business we were still unfamiliar with. I had never managed a set of accounts, done any marketing or even knew what SEO stood for. The difference was I was prepared to learn. I took the same approach that I did when I first started playing poker. I started watching video tutorials on YouTube, I read books on business management, I even bought an online course on marketing.

I was relentless in my aim to be the best I could be. I used to cower from learning something new, whereas now I see it as an opportunity to improve. If I didn't know something that could benefit me, I would make sure that I knew it well enough to teach it. For example I said I know nothing about marketing when I first started. I now run business and marketing days for some of our corporate partners' staff.

Curveball

Everything was going fine until my former employers got in touch claiming that I was breaching a clause in my contract by setting up a business in the same sector as theirs. At first this caused me to panic. It did mentally effect me for a short while, with my work productivity going down as I thought I might have to shut the business down. I was not familiar with legal proceedings and did not know that such a clause even existed. I was not prepared to let my dream slip through my fingers. Instead of sitting in self-pity or simply quitting (like I would have done years ago), I did some research and when I cleared my mind I realised that if what they were saying was right, every hair salon ever started would be closed down. I sought legal help from a solicitor. After consultation with a solicitor I was told my former employers had less than a 1% chance of enforcing any such clause.

Threats

This involved messages from their directors to my company's Facebook page, our chat box on our website and phone calls from withheld numbers followed. They even created a Facebook advert with the promotion code :ORIGYM and changed their entire pricing structure around my company's price. I did the smart thing (I think) and reported them to the governing body and then I thought, I must be doing something right if this is causing them to go to these measures.

I have absolutely no hard feelings towards them and every time they sent a message or tried to provoke a situation I harnessed it as more of an incentive to make this business grow. Even to this day I check their Facebook page and just seeing their logo is enough to make me pick up the laptop and carry on working. I never once wrote back, even when they used their social media platform to insult me personally. I just kept working harder and more frequently to beat them in the long run. The old me would have retaliated in one second flat, that is when I knew my mentality had shifted.

Business Is Booming

This all soon passed and Origym was growing from strength to strength. Students were now completing our course and we were getting fantastic reviews. The governing body even got in touch to ask what strategies we were implementing to generate such large student volumes for a new start up provider. Our first two full time staff members started and we opened up another training venue so that we could hold full time intensive courses as opposed to just online or with a one to one tutor which is what we used initially to scale so fast. Life was good and I was now in the position to take a decent salary home.

Areas Of Weaknesses - Try, Try And Try Again

Some elements of the business were going really well, but other areas started to stagnate. Some of our marketing strategies were not having the same effect that they did before. Our corporate outreach was no longer getting the levels of response and I was getting a little homesick. I had worked for 18 months, having a total of 6 days off in that time period and I was exhausted. I was less productive and my hours were declining through sheer tiredness. So I decided to take a full week off to re-charge. I went back to Birmingham and I did not answer any phone calls or emails during this time as my mind needed to dis-engage from the business. We all need times to recuperate and literally do nothing. Some people say this is unproductive. I disagree. Rest is valuable, only when it becomes 'too much rest' does it become an issue.

As soon as I came back I went straight into the marketing full of fresh ideas. Despite previous setbacks, I systematically employed the same corporate outreach strategy as I knew this had worked in the past, but something before was lacking. I did this against others telling me it did not work and pointing at the minor financial loss we had incurred as a result of this strategy. Sometimes you have to listen to others and not force the issue. But there are times when you have to do what you believe works, which is exactly what I did. Thankfully I did, as it secured my biggest corporate contract to date with one of the UK's largest gym chains.

Hit My Goal

You may be reading and thinking: I thought you wanted to own a gym? I still did even though I loved running the fitness education side of life. I actually bought into Steph's personal training business and at last hit my goal and we were opening our first actual gym on the side of our training facility in Liverpool. It had taken me 3 years and 204 days from day that I had confided in my parents about being unhappy with work and life in general. When I think about it and reel off the list of things I have achieved in that time period, it makes me really proud.

I'm reminded of how far I have come from being someone who was disillusioned with their life to now, where I actually respect myself for what I have done. Don't get me wrong, it is not a miracle or anything absolutely astounding. But it gives me a sense of accomplishment.

Closing Thoughts

Steph and I now own 11 gyms in 10 cities across the UK. The education company graduates around 1200 students per annum, the 5th highest in the UK. We are also launching an additional company at the moment that is also going to compliment the other two.

I am still working as much as ever and I genuinely love getting up in the morning and going to work. Every day I set myself goals and targets towards an overall objective for my business. It truly is the best thing that has ever happened to me. But it has been very hard work, something that I now actually look forward to. I'm always seeking opportunities and never miss a chance if a potential avenue surfaces.   As you probably know by now, I don't have a strong academic background or have a natural intellectual gift. I have a clear goal, I evaluate how I am going to get to that goal and then I take action and work hard. This is the formula that has worked well for me both at work and at home. It gives me inner peace that, no matter what happens, If I fail or succeed I always, always give it my absolute best shot.

Luke Hughes

About The Author

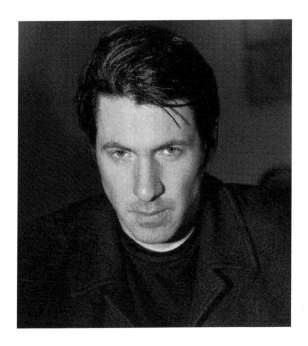

Luke is a serial entrepreneur with business's that focus in the health and fitness sector. He co-founded Origym Centre of Excellence LTD an education company for the fitness sector, Origym LTD, which sells online personal training, clothing and nutritional products and Origym Group LTD which is now the largest group of private fitness studios in the UK with eleven sites UK-wide.

Luke who is originally from Birmingham and now resides in Liverpool, where his business head office is situated, loves trying to play football, poker and of course fitness where the passion for his brand derives.

Origym

WEBSITE: https://origympersonaltrainercourses.co.uk/

FACEBOOK: https://www.facebook.com/origymCOE/

TWITTER: @Origym_COE

Overcoming Any Adversity In Your Life - If I Can You Can

It is said that in order for a child to grow into a healthy, happy and caring adult all they need is the love and support of just one caring adult. Just one person to believe in them; support them in times of need and to help instill good values and beliefs in themselves. But what happens when a child does not have this kind of support system in place can they still become a happy person?

For me I've felt like an outsider my whole life. Someone with orphan energy, the kind of person no one really wanted in their family and, sadly, I actually lacked that one caring adult.

I grew up in a fairly typical environment that changed when I was 12 and my parent's divorced. I loved my dad and had been his shadow for as long as I could remember. So it came as a great shock when my mother was awarded custody of their three youngest children. I was devastated that my father didn't want me.

Trouble was my mother didn't want me either. She only took me in just to spite my father. It was odd at first; you see I had never really bonded with her.

My sister who was 8 years older than me, looked after the needs of both my sister and I and inadvertently she became our mother.

She married a few weeks before my parents split so now I was all alone with this person who was technically my mother, but not really my mum.

When I look back I can't ever remember her ever hugging me and she certainly never told me she loved me. As an adult with my own child I look back and think how terribly odd that was.

A few days after my 13th birthday I had an access visit with my father. He gave me the best birthday present ever - a long sleek black coat. I'd never had anything new like this before (hand me downs was all we could afford) and it was the kind of gift I would treasure forever.

Upon my arrival home I had barely taken my prized possession out of its bag when my mother confiscated it. She rationalized that it was way too extravagant a gift for me to have and decided that since my siblings didn't get luxury gifts from my father I wouldn't either.

A heated argument erupted but my protests fell on deaf ears. Having had enough, she pushed passed me and went out into our backyard. What could she possible do with my coat out there I wondered?

I paused momentarily in disbelief at what I thought she was going to do and therefore didn't get the chance to stop her hurling my beautiful coat into our lit incinerator. Her look of satisfaction equally matched my look of mortification as my coat went up in flames.

I'll never forget the volcano that erupted within me and in that moment ended any chance the two of us ever had at a real mother daughter relationship.

From that day on I made a promise to myself that I would fill her life with as much pain and misery as I experienced on that day.

I don't remember when our agreements turned physical, but I do remember them being loud and often with me being on the receiving end of her beatings.

I'm sure our whole neighbourhood heard us 'go at it.'

Not long before my 15th birthday and after years of being on the receiving end of her physical abuse, I simple stood up for myself and fought back. I'm sure it came as a shock the first time my fist connected with her chin and she was sent reeling.

From that day on our fights were like those memorable boxing matches with Muhammad Ali and his contenders. Some days she was the victor others I was.

I have lots of emotionally charged memories of the two of us throwing punches at each other and I lost count of the number of days I ended up with bruises. I spent many a night recovering at a friend's house before re-entering the battle zone.

I had learnt to become a prolific liar so that people wouldn't know that my mother at 5 foot nothing gave me the bruises I sported on a weekly basis.

Not long after my 18th birthday I landed a job. Instead of coming home to congratulations and the celebrations I thought would ensure I got "well now you can pay board and make my life easier."

A few days later after another heated argument I was banished from my family home forever. And I have to give it to my mother, when she makes a promise she certainly knows how to keep it. Her "I'm never going to talk to you again" reverberates as loudly today as it did 30 years ago. She died in 2015 having never spoken to me again.

Being homeless was a shock to my system. I was fortunate enough to live in a friends' spare room for a while before moving in with my paternal grandmother. I was surprised to find my father also lived there and our relationship picked up right where it left off 6 years earlier.

Fast-forward 30 years and things certainly changed. When I was homeless and the future looked very bleak all I wanted was to be happily married, with kids and a great home. You know the kind of fantasy all girls want. Well it took a lot of hard work, sometimes working two and three jobs to achieve my goals but I did it and would have considered against all odds to be very happy.

Then my father died. It was not his actual death that plagued me into what I call 'my dark days" but a series of events that occurred shortly afterwards.

The arrival of a letter from a solicitor a week after his death set a strange series of events into motion. Being the sole heir and benefactor of my father's modest estate I remember joking with my daughter "poppy must have left us a secret stash of cash." I can't believe how further from the truth I was.

I had always thought I was a good daughter and my father and I had an ok relationship. Often strained by his alcoholism and his emotional out bursts, but I was hell bent on making sure he never felt alone.

I helped him reconnect with his grandchildren (his three other children never spoke to him after my parent's divorce) and organised birthday and Christmas parties to encourage these relationships. We even went away on holidays together and my family and I visited him often.

So you could image my reaction at reading this new will and he equated my value along the same line as my other siblings who all turned their backs on him 30 years ago. That value was nothing - which is exactly what he left us all.

When I read further that he'd never really cared for me, that was the moment my heart broke in two and the words "betrayal" came screaming out.

I felt guttered, bamboozled and angry all at once. Now I know he could do whatever he wanted with his money, but when he willed a house I owned outright to someone other than me, the one I let him live in rent free for 25 years, I wanted to scream "what the hell!"

Tears started rolling down my eyes with thoughts of being stupid, hurt and humiliated all infiltrating at an exponential rate.

Rereading his letter, tears now tumbled like a waterfall, all I could think of was "what had I done to hurt him so" and "why did he turn on me like this."

I guess I wasn't really prepared for the answer but when "you're not worthy" screamed back at me, it was so loud my heart skipped a beat.

In an instant I became explosively angry. I was so angry with myself for picking the wrong side. For years I had felt dejected, hurt and often humiliated about not being considered part of my family and not being invited to family events. But I had rationalized my decisions because I felt I had the love of my father. Standing there in that moment though, well there were no words to describe how I really felt. I was guttered and wanted to throw up.

His rejection cut deep. How deep would only be revealed in the coming days when unanswered questions sent my emotions spiralling out of control. I was looking for answers that weren't forth coming and eventually my low self-esteem and unworthiness issues went into over drive. Over the ensuing days I cried for hours on end.

Logical thinking was hard to come by especially as I should have been mourning the loss of my father instead I was gearing up for a battle over my house. My pride also got in the way as I vainly tried to find proof that my father actually loved me and I was devastated that all I had worked so hard for could be taken away in an instant.

It was agonising. It felt surreal and then a strange hollowness settled over me. An emptiness that's hard to describe. It was then I realised I would have to go into battle alone and that there would be no one standing beside me when I did.

Then my 'Pandora's box' (you know that place you store all your sadness, hurt and anger) exploded and hundreds of unhealed emotions spanning the last 4 decades all came hurling at me.

I not only had to deal with how I felt about my father's rejection, I also had to deal with the many issues from my teenage years including my mother's abuse, becoming the black sheep of my family and the sexual abuse I suffered at the hands of the neighbourhood boys.

At the forefront was the humiliation over my first marriage, which dissolved after only a year, the loss of a lot of money and the loss of an unborn child.

The wounds began to manifest deeper as hundreds of so-called non-events from my past started to show up to help with my 'emotional cleansing.'

At one stage I had so many issues to contemplate I didn't know where to start. Questions kept circulating yet the answers I needed remained elusive. With no support system in place I felt a small piece of my soul die with each passing day.

I felt broken and spent most days lying on the couch crying, unable to function. I eventually stopped eating, stopping communicating with my family and slowly began to lose touch with reality. In order to combat this paralyzing effect I started to build a tall wall around me hoping to keep the pain at bay.

This agony went on for weeks and I was slowly losing the battle.

I remember my daughter coming home from school one day to find me still on the couch in my pyjamas. I'd actually thought she had just left something at home and was mortified to find that 8 hours had actually passed. That was the straw that broke the camel's back.

I was finally beaten. Unable to go on I allowed the darkness that I had been experiencing over the last couple of weeks to fully encapsulated me. I made the painful decision that tomorrow it would all end.

They say that when the student is ready the teacher will arrive. For me my saving grace came in the form of a friend and mentor who rang later that same night. She explained how she had been reading about emotional wellness and had decided to embark on a 12 weeks course that she thought I would benefit from.

An hour later I saw a flicker of hope that maybe there was a way out, but did I have the strength and determination to climb back towards the light. They say life is all about the decisions we make and in that moment I decided the darkness was not my destiny.

One of the very first things Jenny talked about was being responsible for your actions and that on some level you are responsible for what is happening in your life.

I remember thinking that was nonsense. There was no way I had created all the pain and suffering that I was experiencing. My pride wanted me to believe that this was happening to me because of what someone else had done- not because of something I had done.

That was the day my eyes truly opened to the fact that we all create our own reality. On some level when things go wrong we often find it's easier to blame someone else rather than be responsible for the part we may have played in it all. By blaming someone else we don't have to be accountable for our actions.

We've all done it, blamed someone else for what's happened in our lives. I was interested to learn we do so not because we want to hurt others but because we have not yet fully learnt to trust the consequences of our own actions. The FEAR (False Evidence Appearing Real) of the unknown and the final outcome can be quite paralyzing.

When one learns to be fully responsible for their actions then they have the power to effect real change. Real change means the ability to heal the pain of the past. By healing our pain we have the ability to create our own Destiny. This is where I wanted to be heading, but there were be many hurdles to overcome.

So one of the first steps I had to embrace was to learn to be fully accountable for my actions good or bad.

That meant I had to be brutally honest with myself about why I didn't see that my father had an up to date will. Or why I had decided not to get more involved in his care or why I willingly allowed a family friend to care for him when her offer came in. Did I not want to acknowledge he was dying or did I just not care?

The truth can be so liberating and so damn scary at the same time.

Jenny asked me to write down all the issues that had been circling in my head especially the ones that simply had no answers forthcoming. She asked me to assess each situation to see the role I had played.

Getting started terrified me. It was a real wake-up call sifting through the emotional baggage I had been carrying for years. I found that there were two main sections. Issues I created and ones that others created that I had either allowed to happen or was too afraid to speak up about.

Whenever I came across an incident that someone else choreographed I chose to do the *letter writing release*. This is where you simply write the person a letter telling him or her how you felt. You see the objective is not to make the other person wrong but for you to put your point of view across.

Isn't this why we get angry in the first place, walking away from a situation and not having said what it is you wanted to say?

How often have you then thought of the perfect comeback yet it came several hours or even days later, and your chance to say anything long gone? By having your say now gives you the opportunity to allow the incident to come full circle and thus be healed.

At first I thought this was really silly. Then I was surprised to read that your subconscious does not know the difference between what is real and what is imagined. The subconscious operates on commands and time is irrelevant.

I also learned that most of our DOS programming (our internal filters) are instilled in us between the ages of 5- 12 years old. It's these programs that become hardwired and dictate how we live our lives. Often these automated decisions are carried out subconsciously and we may not even be aware of their origins or existence.

That's what I experienced that day I got the solicitor's letter; my automatic response when feeling dejected was anger.

In order to help heal my anger and rid some of my emotional baggage, I had to locate toxic incidents and then rewrite a new ending. With my mother I had a prince rescue me on more than one occasion. Yes, laugh if you must.

Remember that there are no right or wrong answers here. Your subconscious is not judgmental it is designed to just accept what is. So although I could not change what happened I did have the power to change how I felt in any given scenario and that's what

I did. It only had to make sense to me.

In a short period of time I wrote hundreds of letters, some to my parents and siblings and some to people who are no longer on this earth. I even wrote to bystanders that stood around and did not intervene when they should have. I didn't have to send them for the very act of acknowledging how I felt gave me the validation I needed to remove the charge (angst) about the situation. Once your secrets have been aired they no longer hold any power.

With the angst now gone the chances of my subconscious selecting that particular memory and releasing that emotion lessened.

I even wrote letter apologizing to others for my behaviour. The one to my mother left me sobbing uncontrollably for hours.

As each incident came full circle I started feeling lighter as the emotional baggage I had carried for years lifted off my shoulders. (Now I know why confession can be so enlightening.)

Week 3 of Jenny's course found the key that unlocked some of my own DOS programming. We did a word association game and the word *dominated* came up.

I couldn't believe how much this word resonated with me. I cried for hours thinking how I let my father bully me, my mother too. And there were hundreds of other incidents with a bullying theme attached to them. I couldn't believe another program from my childhood had been stuck on replay.

I hadn't realised when memories are created they become impregnated with an emotion. Each time the memory is triggered the attached emotion is activated providing an actions or reactions. For me whenever I felt ignored - anger was my response.

Oddly enough some underlying issues was so subtle I nearly missed it. Take for example how easy it is for programming to take root.

When I was 7 I went to see my mother about something. She was busy in the kitchen and brushed me aside. (Not really but that's how we view incidents through the eyes of a child.) I remember wanting to show her my picture right before dinner—again I got ignored. The third time I tried to get her attention she was cleaning up after dinner. See how unassuming the actions of the parent can be but how the child could easily misinterpret the situation with their childlike vocabulary. Although my mother did nothing wrong I internalized her actions and created a subliminal programming that said "I hate being ignored."

A program that ran for many years, and oddly enough collected other incidents to help validate it, was when I didn't get asked to a party. I felt I was being ignored. I remember asking my daughter to do something and I got angry for I felt I was being ignored. Overlooked for a promotion – ignored again.

Here's the most intriguing piece of info I've uncovered on my journey so far;

Memories do not have a shelf life or good for one use only. It's therefore possible that a toxic memory (me being ignored) has the probability of showing up time and time again. Releasing its charge (my anger) over and over again, even decades later. (Remember the subconscious cannot tell timelines it simply acts on commands. When memories are summoned they simply release the emotion within.)

That's exactly what was happening to me. My highly charged emotions were coming at me thick and fast, especially the ones that had done the rounds year after year after year. These were the ones that were contributing to my outbursts, the ones that were now making my life miserable.

Thankfully I now had the tools to combat my feelings and deactivate these time bombs from ever going off again. It took about 6 weeks for the big issues to dissipate and I am still a work in progress some 7 years later.

They say tears are a great way to cleanse the soul and I knew from the amount I have cried that I must have been releasing and shifting something within me.

I once heard a phrase that I love to use: *if nothing changes – nothing changes.*

It takes real courage to step into the unknown and go "yep that's for me." I once had a teacher tell me "some people would rather stay in their comfort zone and be miserable than to venture out and see what's possible."

For me I'd had enough of misery.

Was it hard? Absolutely, but not impossible. I believe that you are your own destiny. You get to be the bus driver of your life. If you don't like where you are heading only you can make the necessary decisions to change. Altering ones course though can be awfully taxing.

I could be angry with all that happened, but I have to believe that there was a bigger picture in play. For me I had to go through this excruciating pain and suffering to come out the other end a different person.

I now understand that although we need the love of a parent to get us started in life our ultimate goal is to learn how to self-love. Something most of us have no real idea how to do, so we spend a lifetime relying on others to fill the void that we have deep within. I fully understand now that we get back in abundance what we send out. If you are miserable then more will come your way. If you are happy then the Universe will send more for you to be happy about.

Self-love is the true key to happiness and its available to those willing to go the distance.

Along my journey I found other pieces of wisdom that I want to share with you in order to make your journey of self-discovery a little smoother.

1. We all have *a story* about what someone did or didn't do to us. Often we can become the story for why we do not have the

success we had hoped to achieve in life. For me, the violence in my childhood allowed me to think I was not good enough. And although I have had some success in my life I chose to aim for the roof instead of the stars. Fear of failing made me play safe.

2. We all lie. Even white lies can prevent you from living an authentic life. Trouble is we've all learned to accept white lies. Those we tell others but more importantly the ones we tell ourselves. Excuses are really just lies we tell ourselves. Being authentic in all we do starts with the truth.

3. Playing above the line is the first step in being responsible for your actions. Imagine a line in the sand and at the top is love and at the bottom fear. When you lie, blame others or justify your life you fall below the line and operate from a level of fear. When you are authentic, tell the truth and own your actions you move above the line towards love.

There will be days when you fall below the line of responsibility. These are the days you dust yourself off, be gentle on yourself and start over. The more you do this the easier it becomes to operate above the line. Operating here is where your personal power lies. No longer will life get to push you around for you now have the controls to make magic happen.

4. Setting good boundaries. How often do you move the goal posts just to accommodate someone else's needs? We all do it. This subliminal programming was started by our parents trying to keep the peace but then become our own mantra. "Why don't you share?" " Stop that" or "don't do that" are among my favorite

comments. It's these kinds of comments that lead us to believe that it is wrong to put our own needs and wants first. It may have served us in our childhood, but as adults if we are not happy, how are we supposed to make those around us happy?

The first step in self-love is to set good boundaries. A good boundary tells people this is how I like to be treated and that I matter.

5. The art of saying no. Another program instilled by our well-meaning parents in order to assert control by making us feel it's wrong to say no.

How often were you made to share a toy or food or told to do something that you didn't want to? Again your feelings were overlooked in order to keep the peace.

Eventually you learn to put your wants and needs to one side and you start to do things to please those around you. Mums are very good at placing themselves last on the family ladder.

Over time we learn to say yes even to things we don't really want to do in order to keep the peace. Then we spend hours or even days looking for an excuse (which is really a lie) in order to negate the offer.

Why do we find it so hard to just say no?

Often it's because we equate a no, with a form of rejection. Remember how hurtful it was as a child not to get your own way, or to not be included. Therefore people say yes even though they really want to scream no.

I use to be a yes person all the time. I now understand that saying no does not mean I am selfish. It just means I love myself enough to put my own needs first, something that is very alien to most of us and takes some practicing to get used to.

Therefore I have the following that I use when asked to go somewhere or do something that is not to my liking. Being so direct can be uncomfortable but persistence pays off.

a. Thank you for thinking of me, but truly that's not for me.
b. I would but I have another appointment or engagement, but I would love to catch up for coffee the next day to see how it all went.
c. I love how we have different tastes but on this occasion that event or occasion does not suit me, but please think of me next time.

Yes the person may be hurt but remind them that you are rejecting the event not them as a person. Always finish with that. When a person realizes that they are not being personally rejected a true friend would understand. If a friend pressures you then maybe you should maybe rethink that relationship.

6. Know what makes you tick. Can you write 10 things that you like to do? Most people I know can do a list of 5 or 6 things but 10 is really tricky. Now every day indulge yourself a little in one or all of those things. Over time learn to build on them. Happy people have interests outside of home and work and can say no to the things they do not like. This then frees up time to indulge

in passions that you like, with the end result you being just that little bit happier.

Change is never easy. Especially when we run into our outdated programming on a daily basis. Everyone has a story but we also have the ability to change the ending to that story. Some take on the challenge and others don't and remain stuck in their programming. Remember I went from being emotionally and physically abused in my youth, to teetering on the poverty line, being homeless and so many other adversities stacked up against me that I was destined to fail - but I didn't.

I learnt to power ahead even when I didn't know where I was headed or what was to come. I now believe that when things don't go as planned, maybe a bigger picture is in play and sometimes we have to take a different course for it to be revealed to us. For me did I really have to go through all this pain and suffering to find inner happiness? Well apparently so and now I help others find the light they need on their journey of self-discovery.

When one learns to ask the right questions, the right tools magically appear and that's when we become the master of our own destiny.

It worked for me and if I can, you can.

Leann Middlemass

About The Author

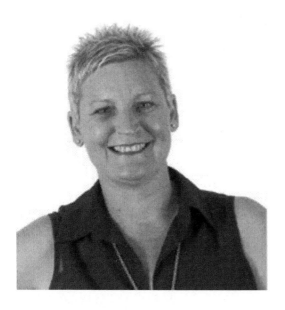

Leann Middlemass is a teacher of Emotional Wellness. Leann spent 10 years studying under Robert Kiyosaki (author of Rich Dad Poor Dad) and went on to use many of Robert's techniques to become a property consultant and self-managed super fund advisor.

Leann is passionate in teaching financial literacy and ran and attended hundreds of seminars on wealth creation. Leann also "wrote and produced an audio called: **"How To Start & Manage Your Own Super Fund"**.

In 2009 Leann suffered a near mental breakdown that drastically changed the direction of her life. The pain and suffering she experienced brought her to the brink of suicide. Her story is one of courage and success.

Leann now teaches other just how powerful emotional baggage is and how although formed in your childhood can still play havoc in your adult life.

Leann's passion is to teach other how to remove this baggage, how to stop others and life from pushing you around and how simple empowerment techniques can allow you to be the master of your own Destiny.

mydestiny.net.au

If I Can, You Can